# Quick & Easy
# Low
# Calorie
## COOKBOOK

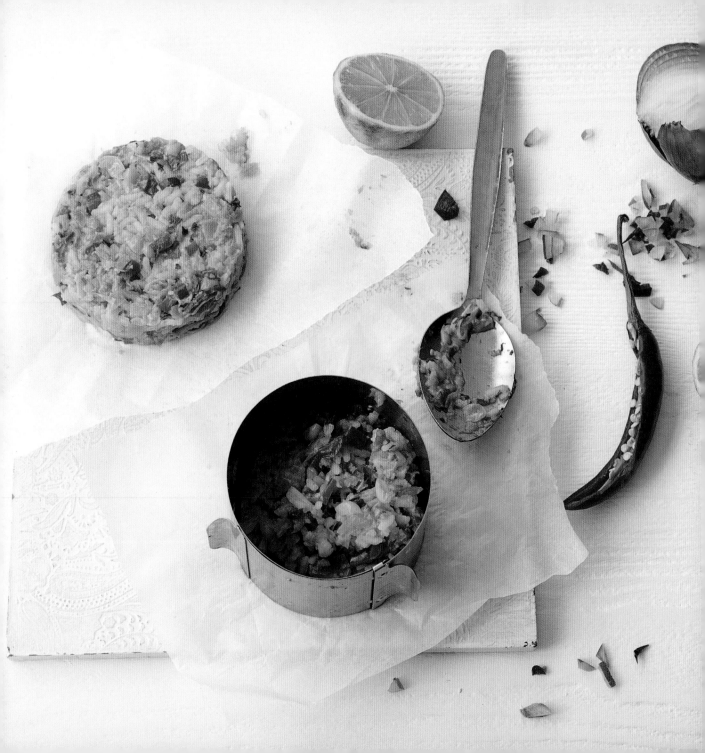

# Quick & Easy Low Calorie COOKBOOK

Heather Thomas

PAVILION

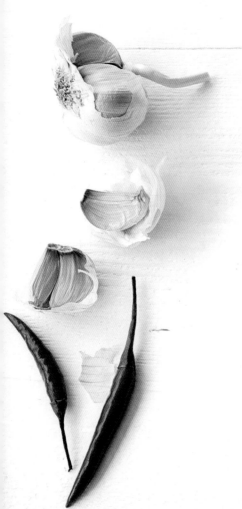

# Contents

Introduction                          006
Slimming success                      008
The 10 commandments                   010
Clever cook                           012
What can I eat?                       014
Healthy flavourings                   016
'Traffic light' foods                 018
Basic recipes                         021

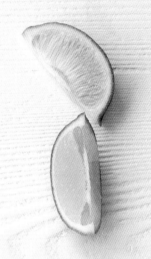

**100 calories**                    **024**

**200 calories**                    **062**

**300 calories**                    **114**

Index                               174

# introduction

The key to losing weight effectively is a regime that's easy to follow, enjoyable, never leaves you feeling hungry and allows you to make your own choices about what to eat. This book takes the guesswork and arithmetic out of calorie counting. Whether you are on a weight-loss programme for just want to maintain your ideal weight, these quick and easy recipes enable you to watch your calorie intake while eating tasty meals that will leave you feeling fuller for longer. You can navigate your way through the day without worrying about calories and quantities – there's no number crunching.

### No guesswork… no counting

No matter what diet you are following or what your daily calorie target is, it's easy to achieve and to stay on course with this book. Throw away your calculator and stop worrying about food – just relax and enjoy every meal. There's no need to guess, because all the recipes fall into 100- , 200- and 300-calorie portions, making weight loss, control and maintenance so easy.

### It works with so many diets

No matter how much or how little weight you have to lose or which diet you are following, this approach works. Whether you are just limiting your daily calorie intake to a specific number per day, dieting online, going to classes or following the 5:2 regime, this book can help and inspire you, making slimming so much simpler. There is no magic formula to dieting – successful weight loss and maintenance are all about calories: how many you consume and how many you burn, and to lose weight you need to take in fewer calories than you use up. Nearly all diets are based on calorie counting, whether they call them by their name or use other systems. When you are in control of the calories you eat, it's easier to manage your weight loss and see the results as the excess pounds and inches disappear.

### What are calories?

Whether you want to lose weight or maintain your ideal weight, it comes down to a simple formula: the calories you consume (from the food you eat) must not exceed the calories you burn in the course of a day – doing chores, working, exercising and going through your daily routine. If we eat more calories than we use, they are stored in our bodies as fat. There are approximately 3,500 calories (or kilocalories/kcals) in 450g/1lb of fat. Therefore to lose a pound, you need to eat 3,500 fewer calories or use them up by exercising – or a combination of both. A calorie is a unit of heat energy that fuels our bodies; high-fat and high-sugar foods contain more calories than those that are low in fat and sugar: you get about 9 calories from 1g fat and about 4 calories from 1g protein.

**Be calorie aware**
By learning about the calorie content of the foods you eat, you can make informed and conscious choices and be more in control of your weight. Always check the labels on foods such as breakfast cereals, ready meals, sauces and salsas, fruit juice and smoothies – although many of them are perceived as healthy, they can contain 'hidden' or 'empty' calories in the form of fat and sugar. And lots of the snack foods that we grab without thinking are loaded with calories. For example, a large caffe latte made with whole milk might contain as many as 225 calories, while a blueberry muffin could add up to 550 calories. Together, that's approximately half the calories people would aim to eat in a day on a 1500 calorie-controlled weight-loss diet!

**Portion control made easy**
In this book you can mix and match your meals to achieve your calorie target each day without agonizing about piling on the pounds – everything is counted for you and portion-controlled to help you manage your weight more effectively. Just choose delicious recipes from the following calorie bands:

**100-calorie breakfasts, brunches, light meals and desserts**
**200-calorie breakfasts, brunches, packed lunches, light meals and desserts**
**300-calorie breakfasts, lunches and main meals**

By taking control of what you eat, you will be more calorie aware as well as feeling healthier and trimmer. You can proceed at your own pace and enjoy a wide range of nutritious foods, including many of your favourites. A lot of calorie-counted diets are complicated and confusing, but we have calculated everything for you in simple round numbers, and all the recipes have fat and fibre counts, so you can make your own choices on what to eat.

**Stay slim**
When you reach your weight-loss goal, you can use the recipes to maintain your ideal weight in the long term. As they are simple to make and taste so good, you will be happy to use them again and again. By adopting a healthier diet and working with simple calorie bands, you will be less likely to regain the weight you have lost. If you have a minor lapse or indulgence, don't worry or feel guilty – just reduce your calorie intake for a day or two and you will be back on track.

# Slimming success

**If you want to be successful at losing weight and staying trim in the long term, you need to learn new healthy eating habits and make them an intrinsic part of your lifestyle. By eating a varied low-fat, low-sugar diet that supplies all the essential nutrients your body needs for good health, you can enjoy your food and never feel hungry. Here are some guidelines to get you going:**

### Don't obsess about your weight
If you get stressed about your weight and how slowly the pounds are dropping off, it will be self-defeating. Successful weight loss is a gradual process and takes time; if you lose weight too fast, you are more likely to put it on again and there may be risks to your health. Don't keep weighing yourself – once a week is enough. Your weight fluctuates from day to day, so you won't get a true picture of how much you have lost.

### Plan ahead
Try not to think too much about food and what you are going to cook for dinner tonight or lunch tomorrow. By planning ahead and doing one big shop instead of making several visits to the supermarket, you can get on with your life and focus on other things. By selecting meals from the 100-, 200- and 300-calorie recipes in this book, it's easy to plan a whole week's menus in advance. By ordering your weekly food online and having it delivered to your home, you are less likely to succumb to the many tempting high-calorie foods you spot as you stroll along the supermarket aisles.

### Feel fuller for longer
By eating high-fibre and low-GI (glycaemic index) foods, such as vegetables, fruit, beans, pulses and oatmeal that are relatively low in calories and release energy slowly, you will feel fuller for longer, help keep your blood glucose and insulin levels stable, and reduce hunger pangs between meals. GI ratings are given for every recipe throughout this book.

### Check food labels carefully
When you are shopping, check the nutritional information on food labels carefully to make sure that even supposedly healthy foods (e.g. smoothies and yogurts) are not high in sugar and fat.

### Recognize your trigger foods
We all have favourite foods and snacks that we love so much that we find it hard to eat them in moderation. They might be sweets (candy), chocolate bars, wine or biscuits (cookies). By acknowledging your weaknesses, you are taking control of what you eat. You can still continue to enjoy them as an occasional treat and within the context of your daily and weekly calorie target.

### Eating out
Just because you're watching your weight doesn't mean that you have to stop eating out. You just need to make sensible choices and know which are the low-calorie healthier options on restaurant menus. As a general rule, salads, grilled food,

fish, seafood and chicken without creamy sauces are the best choices. Pasta is best with a tomato-based sauce rather than a creamy one and you should avoid fried food. Remember that a 125ml/4 fl oz/½ cup glass of dry white wine has 82 calories.

### Drink lots of water

We all need to drink plenty of water every day to stay hydrated and healthy, but drinking a glass of water before a meal can help to fill you up, making it less likely that you will over-eat. Always drink water in preference to sugary soft drinks – it has zero calories. If you are still hungry… have a salad or serve some extra steamed, boiled, grilled or raw vegetables with your meal.

### Set yourself a daily target

Most weight-loss plans set a daily calorie total, which includes breakfast, lunch and dinner, a skimmed (lowfat) milk allowance for hot drinks and cereal, plus a couple of healthy treats. For women, this is usually between 1,200 and 1,400 calories (instead of 1,800–1,900 for normal daily maintenance) and for men it's 1,800 to 1,900 calories (rather than the usual recommended 2,500 required to maintain a healthy body weight). The round number calorie-counted dishes in this book make this easy for you.

### Speed up your weight loss

Instead of eating even less to lose weight more quickly, start exercising to burn up extra calories and slimline your body. You need to exercise for at least 30 minutes four or five times a week. If you choose something you enjoy, you are more likely to stick with it and make it part of your way of life. Join a gym, power walk, go for a jog, cycle or swim, whatever takes your fancy, but don't overdo it. Like dieting, you have to start slowly and build up gradually as you get fitter. If you have any health issues, check with your doctor first.

### Last but not least…

Don't crash diet. You might lose a lot of weight fast initially but you will soon pile it all back on again when you go back to your old eating habits – this is especially true of fad diets that forbid a whole range of essential foods. You need to make long-term changes to your eating habits to lose weight slowly, safely and steadily and keep it off for good.

### Keep a record

Recording what you eat on a daily basis and how much weight you lose per week can be very illuminating when charting your weight-loss progress over a period of weeks or even months. It can also inspire and motivate you if you reach a plateau where the pounds are rolling off more slowly. You may find it helpful to write down the exercise you do, too. Record it in a pocket book or on your smartphone, tablet or computer.

# The 10 commandments

**To use the recipes in this book effectively and to lose weight gradually or maintain your ideal weight, here's a set of 10 basic rules to follow:**

### 1 Eat a varied diet
To stay healthy, you need to eat a varied diet that contains all the essential nutrients: protein (animal and/or vegetable), carbohydrates that are not over-refined or high in sugar, fat (we all need some fat, but choose foods if possible that have less than 5 per cent fat and remove any visible fat from meat and poultry), vitamins and minerals. Even when you are on a calorie-reduced programme, you can still include all these foods on a daily basis. It's particularly important to eat some protein every day because it's needed for body growth and maintenance, building muscle and repairing damaged tissue. Good sources are chicken, turkey, lean beef, pork and lamb, white and oily fish, shellfish, eggs, beans, pulses, whole grains, nuts, soy and low-fat dairy products, such as skimmed (lowfat) milk and very low-fat yogurt.

### 2 Eat three meals a day
You must eat three meals a day – breakfast, lunch and dinner – that fit within your daily calorie target. Eating regularly within a routine that suits you and your lifestyle makes you less likely to feel hungry between meals or to get sugar cravings. Many people are tempted to skip breakfast and just have a coffee, but this is a big mistake and counter-productive. Eating breakfast raises your blood sugar levels after a night's sleep and boosts your metabolism so your body is less sluggish and burns up more calories. If you don't eat breakfast, you are more likely to get hunger pangs as the morning progresses and to snack on high-calorie foods.

### 3 Don't starve yourself
If you go without food and miss meals, you will just crave it even more and be tempted to eat high-calorie foods that put on weight. There's no excuse for skipping meals or reducing your calorie intake to zilch. Within this book, you will find lots of exciting and innovative recipes for low-calorie dishes you can eat and enjoy without worrying about how they are going to affect your weight. If you stop eating, your metabolism will slow down, you will feel weak and less energetic and your health will suffer.

### 4 Try not to snack
If you eat regular healthy meals, you are less likely to snack in between. Most people grab a chocolate bar, a packet of crisps (potato chips), a biscuit (cookie), a cake or sugary drink as a snack, but these will pile on the calories. If you are hungry, it's much better to treat yourself to some fresh fruit, such as an apple, pear, juicy peach or apricot, orange, a slice of melon or some strawberries. Avoid bananas, as they are very starchy and even a small one contains 90 calories and a large one as much as 180 calories. Or you could try a 0% fat plain Greek yogurt with some fresh berries. Healthy vegetable snacks include celery sticks or sliced carrot or red and yellow (bell) pepper with reduced-fat tomato salsa or a small ramekin of virtually fat-free fromage frais sprinkled with chopped fresh herbs. Or spread some low-fat cottage cheese or low-fat hummus on a crispbread and top with some sliced tomato or cucumber.

### 5 Eat less sugar
Sugar is empty calories and doesn't contribute nutritionally to building and maintaining good health. The problem is

that most of us have a sweet tooth and we crave sugar – hence our consumption of biscuits (cookies), cake, desserts, sweet breakfast cereals, ice cream and chocolate. And there are hidden sugars in many sauces, sweetened yogurts, soft drinks, flavoured waters and even coleslaw. Alcohol is probably the worst culprit and if you enjoy a glass or two of wine with your meal every evening, the calories soon add up over the weeks and months. You can reduce your sugar intake by choosing sugarless or low-sugar foods and drinks and using an artificial sweetener or a natural one, such as stevia, in hot drinks.

## 6 Eat less fat

Fat is packed with more calories than any other food, so it's important to keep it to a minimum. You can do this by choosing low-fat foods with less than 5 per cent fat, such as minced (ground) beef, yogurt, ice cream and cottage cheese. Don't spread butter on bread, toast and crispbreads; choose lean cuts of meat and remove all the visible fat before cooking; use spray oil and fat-free vinaigrette dressing and grill, steam or poach foods rather than frying them. Chicken and other poultry and game are naturally lean, but the skin is high in fat, so remove it before cooking if possible, or cut it off roasted birds and discard. However, don't cut out oily fish, such as salmon, mackerel and tuna, which are high in healthy omega-3 fatty acids – try to eat them once or twice a week.

## 7 Eat more fibre

The natural fibre in food not only helps to fill you up so you don't want to eat so much, it also helps keep your gut healthy and your digestive system working efficiently. Vegetables, fruit, whole grains, beans and pulses are all good sources of fibre and you should try to include some of them in your diet every day.

## 8 Eat fewer processed foods

By eating more natural and less refined foods, you will know which nutrients and how many calories they contain. Sugar and fats often lurk in processed foods, sometimes hiding behind other names (see pages 19–20). You don't have to decipher the labels and consume non-nutritious additives, such as flavour enhancers, colourings and preservatives. You are more in control of what you're eating.

## 9 Be aware of hidden calories

Alcohol, canned and fresh soups, sauces, ketchup, mayonnaise and breakfast cereals, including granola, are some of the foods that contain 'hidden' calories. For example, a typical can of soft drink might have the equivalent of as many as 7 teaspoons of sugar. And there are 'hidden' fats in many naturally healthy foods, such as peanuts (5 calories per nut), olives (between 3 and 9 calories each) and avocados (between 200 and 400 calories depending on its size).

## 10 Allow yourself the occasional treat

Just because you are watching the calories and trying to lose weight doesn't mean that you can't indulge yourself with the odd treat. There's no need to feel guilty – we all need to spoil ourselves sometimes. If you achieve the goals you have set and then reward yourself with a treat, that's motivating. Enjoying a sweet food that you crave can help you to stay on track rather than giving up on your weight-loss regime. Just remember to add it to your daily calorie total.

# Clever cook

Cooking should be enjoyable, not a chore, so keep it simple. If you have the right utensils and use healthy cooking methods, cooking the low-fat way is easy. When you are on a diet, you don't want to be agonizing and thinking about food all the time or spending too long in the kitchen where there are so many temptations, and that's why most of the recipes in this book are so quick and easy.

## Cooking the low-fat way

Instead of frying and roasting food in butter and oil, get used to cooking without the extra fat and calories – it's not difficult and it will taste just as good. It's important to have the right pans and equipment to make the whole process easier for you. You will need the following:

- A ridged griddle or grill pan for grilling meat, chicken, fish, seafood and vegetables as well as halloumi cheese and heating tortillas and wraps.
- A few non-stick, sturdy good-quality saucepans in a range of sizes with thick bases, lids and ovenproof handles.
- A non-stick wok (or one that has been properly seasoned so that food will not stick to it and you won't need more than a quick spray of oil) or a non-stick deep frying pan for stir-fries and searing chicken and steaks.
- A small non-stick frying pan for omelettes, frittatas and tortillas.
- A flameproof casserole dish and some baking dishes.
- Some non-stick roasting pans and baking trays.
- Blender and/or food processor for blitzing soups, dressings and dips and making smoothies.

When you are cooking with less fat, you need to ensure that the food stays moist and appetizing. For example, don't over-cook grilled and roasted fish, chicken and meat, or it will start to dry out and lose its succulent tenderness.

Here's some essential information on the cooking methods and techniques you can use to stay healthy and reduce your calorie intake:

## Measuring spoons

A set of standard measuring spoons is an incredibly useful kitchen tool. Not only are they invaluable when adding spices, they can also avoid guesswork – and save calories – when you add a tablespoonful of yogurt or grated Parmesan to top a sweet or savoury dish.

### Non-stick pans

The great thing about non-stick pans is that you can use less fat (oil and butter) when you are cooking. They are safe to use as long as you don't overheat them to the extent that the coating starts to break down and decompose. When this happens, throw the pan away and buy a new one. Always remember to use a wooden spoon, not a metal one, when stirring so as not to scratch the surface.

### Grilling

Whether you use an overhead grill, a griddle pan or a barbecue, grilling uses minimal oil and it's very fast. Lightly spray the pan or the barbecue with oil (you need only one or two sprays) and let it get very hot before adding the food. Sear chicken and meat on both sides over a high heat to stop the juices escaping and to get a good browned flavour and then cook for the recommended time on a slightly lower heat. If you are using an overhead grill, brush the food with a little marinade or spray lightly with oil before cooking. Vegetables can be chargrilled very successfully and using a ridged pan will leave attractive stripes on courgettes (zucchini), aubergines (eggplants) and (bell) peppers.

### Baking and roasting

Use the minimum of oil for roasting vegetables, chicken, meat and fish – just a light spray. Check and turn the food occasionally so it cooks evenly. If it seems to be drying out, you can add a spoonful of stock to moisten it or even some lemon juice.

### Poaching

You can poach chicken, salmon and other fish in some water or stock in a saucepan on the stove or in a covered baking dish in the oven. This cooking method retains the food's natural moisture and prevents it drying out.

### Steaming

It's worth investing in a steamer basket to place above a saucepan of simmering water. Steaming vegetables keeps them slightly crunchy and preserves their nutrients as well as their colour and natural flavours. It's a very healthy way to cook fish and shellfish, too.

### Stir-frying

You need only a couple of sprays of oil to cook a complete meal in a wok. The trick is to place the wok over a high heat and use foods that have been chopped into small pieces so they cook through quickly. Keep stirring all the time so the food does not stick. Flavour it with stock, soy sauce or Thai fish sauce just before serving. This is the quickest and easiest cooking method of all.

### Dry-frying

If you use a preheated non-stick pan set over a medium heat, you can dry-fry meat and chicken without any oil. Sear it on all sides in the hot pan and then reduce the heat immediately before adding vegetables and other ingredients. You can cook low-fat minced (ground) meat in this way, too. When it releases its fat, strain it off through a colander or sieve and then wipe out the pan with some kitchen paper before returning the meat to it or adding onions and other vegetables. You can also dry-fry vegetables, but you may need to add a tablespoon or two of stock to keep them moist and stop them drying out.

### Oil spray

Many of the recipes in this book use spray oil – for grilling, frying and roasting. A tablespoon of oil or butter comes in at around 120 calories, so spray oil can save hundreds of calories every time you cook. You can buy 'one-calorie' oil sprays, or simply fill a spray bottle with olive oil and use to lightly spray a non-stick pan before heating it.

# What can I eat?

**The simple answer to this question is that whether you are trying to drop a dress size or shift several pounds, you can enjoy a very varied diet, which is full of vegetables, fruit, meat, poultry, fish and low-fat dairy products, as well as moderate amounts of breads, pasta, noodles, rice and other grains, the occasional sweet treat. This book is packed with quick, easy, low-calorie versions of many of your favourite meals. On pages 18–20 you will find a detailed 'traffic lights' guide to what you can eat freely, what to eat in small quantities or occasionally, and what to avoid.**

### Get stocked up

Below are some general guidelines on staples to keep in your kitchen cupboard, refrigerator and freezer. With these foods to hand, you will never have an excuse not to cook a slimming meal – there will be plenty of food and you won't have to make daily trips to the supermarket for ready meals or order high-calorie takeaways.

### Choose low-fat dairy

Get into the habit of buying low-fat dairy foods, such as very low-fat or 0% fat plain yogurt. Check the nutritional information on pots of fruit yogurt carefully – many that are low in fat contain a lot of added sugar and are quite high in

> ### Ready meals
>
> If you really don't have time to cook and have to resort to the odd ready meal, keep a few healthy low-calorie ones in the freezer just in case. Choose complete meals of less than 400 calories per serving and serve with salad or green vegetables.

calories. Always buy skimmed (lowfat) milk to use in tea and coffee and on breakfast cereals, to make white sauces and pancakes (crêpes). Experiment with low-fat cheeses, such as Quark, cottage cheese and virtually fat-free fromage frais. If you must use cream, choose half-fat crème fraîche and use only in moderation. When buying hard cheeses, try reduced-fat Cheddar, mozzarella and feta – they are all suitable for cooking.

### Switch to low-fat foods

Look for low-fat versions of the foods you tend to eat regularly, such as extra light mayonnaise; oil-free salad dressings; low-fat ice cream; low-fat minced (ground) beef and lamb (less than 5% fat); reduced-fat coconut milk; and even Quorn vegetarian products. When grilling, shallow-frying and stir-frying, instead of oil, coconut oil or butter, always use a spray oil (see box on page 13).

### Cut your sugar consumption

While cutting down on fat will undoubtedly save calories, many 'low-fat' versions of favourite foods such as biscuits (cookies), ice cream, sauces and dressings are high in sugar: it pays to read the labels when you buy processed foods. The calories in sugar are 'empty' – in other words, they do not contribute to good health – and excess sugar consumption is linked to many long-term health problems, from obesity and type 2 diabetes to hardening of the arteries and premature skin ageing, not to mention dental decay. And sugar is addictive, as you will know if you suffer from cravings for sweet food. Fruits are high in natural sugar, but they bring the benefits of vitamins and minerals, so crunch out your craving with a carrot or a juicy apple, or quench it with a refreshing grapefruit or a glass of fizzy mineral water flavoured with a good squeeze of lemon or lime juice. The calories in that glass of wine – even though it doesn't taste sweet – are also from sugars. So make sure your occasional treats are just that – a treat, once or twice a week.

## Refresh your refrigerator
Keep a range of healthy and low-calorie foods you like to eat and cook with in your refrigerator. Here are some suggestions for the basics:
- Skimmed (lowfat) milk and low-fat yogurts
- Free-range eggs
- Mineral water and diet/zero/low-cal drinks
- Thai green and red curry sauce
- Extra-light mayonnaise
- Dijon mustard
- Oil-free vinaigrette dressing
- Reduced-fat cheese, e.g. mozzarella or Cheddar
- Cottage cheese and virtually fat-free fromage frais
- Tofu, Quorn
- Tzatziki, reduced-fat tomato salsa and pesto, low-fat hummus
- Salad leaves, cucumber, (bell) peppers, tomatoes
- Onions, garlic, carrots, celery
- Green vegetables
- Fresh ginger, chillies, lemongrass
- Lemons and limes
- Fresh herbs

## Top up the freezer
You can freeze clearly labelled individual portions of soups, stews, casseroles, curries, pasta sauces, home-made stock, etc., plus the following:
- Frozen raw prawns (shrimp)
- Frozen seafood
- Chicken breasts
- Low-fat ice cream
- Herbs
- Frozen peas
- Frozen berries
- Sliced wholegrain bread (just use one slice at a time and use the defrost button on the toaster)
- Tortillas and pitta breads
- Filo pastry (dough)

### Packed lunches
If you have a well-stocked refrigerator, freezer and storecupboard, you will always be able to prepare a delicious packed lunch, whether it's a salad or a sandwich. Take a pitta bread or wrap and fill with drained canned tuna, extra-light mayonnaise, some tomato, cucumber and lettuce. If you are out and about and need to grab some food on the go, carefully check the labels on ready-made sandwiches and salads and choose ones with less than 350 calories.

## Stock up your storecupboard with these useful staples and flavourings:
- Canned beans, e.g. butter (lima) beans, chickpeas, cannellini, haricot and kidney beans
- Canned tomatoes and passata (strained tomatoes)
- Canned tuna in spring water
- Jars of capers, gherkins and roasted (bell) pepper strips
- Tabasco, harissa and sweet chilli sauce
- Soy sauce, oyster sauce and nam pla (Thai fish sauce)
- Reduced-fat coconut milk
- Red wine, white wine and cider vinegars
- Good-quality aged balsamic vinegar
- Spray oil
- Brown rice, risotto rice, basmati rice
- Pasta, e.g. soup pasta, spaghetti, linguine, fettuccine, vermicelli, fusilli
- Rice noodles, Chinese egg noodles
- Couscous, bulgur wheat, quinoa
- Sea salt and black peppercorns
- Dried chillies and herbs, spices and seasonings (see pages 16–17)
- Stock cubes (vegetable, chicken, beef) or vegetable bouillon powder
- Dried porcini mushrooms
- Prunes and dried apricots
- Cocoa, baking powder, flour and cornflour
- Porridge (rolled) oats and oatmeal
- Artificial sweeteners and low-calorie sugar substitutes, such as Half-Spoon
- Low-calorie crispbreads, rice cakes

# Healthy flavourings

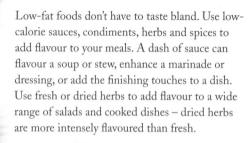

Low-fat foods don't have to taste bland. Use low-calorie sauces, condiments, herbs and spices to add flavour to your meals. A dash of sauce can flavour a soup or stew, enhance a marinade or dressing, or add the finishing touches to a dish. Use fresh or dried herbs to add flavour to a wide range of salads and cooked dishes – dried herbs are more intensely flavoured than fresh.

## Basics

Balsamic vinegar: this is an excellent fat-free salad dressing. Don't buy the cheapest – opt for an aged, syrupy full-flavoured one. Sprinkle over salads, vegetables, chicken and even strawberries.

Lemon and lime: the grated zest and juice will add a fresh, tart citrus flavour to salads, grilled chicken, fish and vegetables.

Mustard: stir into salad dressings, marinades and glazes for meat, but use only sparingly.

Pepper: grind whole peppercorns fresh. Available as black, white or even pink – black has the most pungent flavour.

Salt: sea salt is best, either coarse crystals (flakes) or finely ground. Use sparingly and taste the food before adding salt to any dish.

Stock cubes: add to soups and casseroles or to the vegetable cooking water. Use vegetable, porcini and chicken cubes.

## Sauces

Harissa paste: a hot aromatic chilli paste from North Africa. Serve with couscous, tagines, lamb or chicken kebabs and other Moroccan dishes.

Nam pla (Thai fish sauce): this is a very strong-smelling salty sauce used in Thai curries, stir-fries and dressings.

Oyster sauce: a low-calorie sauce used to flavour Chinese vegetable, chicken or beef stir-fries.

Soy sauce: a salty Asian sauce; add a few drops to stir-fries, gravies and casseroles. Sprinkle over rice or use with lime juice, coriander (cilantro) and chilli as a dip or salad dressing.

Sweet chilli sauce: add a teaspoonful to Asian salad dressings or serve with stir-fries and grilled chicken. Drizzle over low-fat fromage frais as a dip for vegetable crudités.

Tabasco: this is a fiery red chilli sauce, to be used sparingly. Add just a dash to enhance soups or cottage pie.

Teriyaki: use this Japanese sauce to marinate chicken and salmon. It's quite salty, so go easy.

Worcestershire sauce: adds piquancy to soups, stews and casseroles; good with meat.

## Herbs

Basil: this is used in Mediterranean cooking, especially with tomatoes, in salads and pasta sauces. It is also blitzed with oil, pine nuts and garlic to make pesto. Thai basil has a sweet flavour and is used widely in Asian dishes.

Bay leaf: an aromatic leaf of the bay tree used to flavour soups, stews, casseroles, bread sauce and in bouquet garni (a tied bundle of parsley, bay leaf and thyme), it is available fresh or dried.

Chives: best used fresh and snipped with scissors over salads or used as a garnish. Chives have a mild oniony flavour.

Coriander (cilantro): a very distinctive flavour that you love or hate. It is used widely in Asian and Mexican cooking to enhance spicy food. You can eat the leaves and stalks.

Dill: a delicate feathery herb that complements white and oily fish. Use fresh.

Fennel: feathery leaves with a mild aniseed flavour, it is usually used with fish.

Garlic: versatile, aromatic and pungent, garlic has many health-benefits and adds flavour to the blandest ingredients; use sparingly in most dishes. Garlic salt, garlic chives and wild garlic leaves are also available.

Kaffir lime leaves: these fragrant leaves are used fresh or dried in Thai and Asian cooking. They have a citrusy taste.

Marjoram: this herb is used fresh or dried, often in tomato-based sauces, and has a delicate flavour.

Mint: there are many varieties of mint available, including spearmint and peppermint. Add to salads, tabbouleh, tzatziki and lamb. Best used fresh.

Oregano: Has a stronger flavour than marjoram. Add to tomato sauces, salads, aubergine (eggplant) dishes and lamb. Parsley: this herb comes in flat-leaf and curly varieties. It is used to flavour a wide range of dishes.

Rosemary: intensely aromatic, bittersweet-flavoured leaves, rosemary is good with grilled meats and vegetables. The stripped woody stems can be used as 'skewers' for kebabs.

Sage: an aromatic bitter herb. Used in stuffings for poultry and pork, Italian dishes and to flavour soups and casseroles.

Thyme: sweet flavoured tiny leaves, used in soups, casseroles, stuffings and to flavour chicken, pork, lamb and Mediterranean dishes.

## Spices

Allspice: also called pimento or Jamaican pepper, it is available as whole dried berries or ground into powder. It adds an aromatic taste to sweet and savoury dishes, especially jerked chicken.

Cayenne: a fiery red powder, this is used in curries or to sprinkle over grilled meat and baked gratins, such as cauliflower cheese.

Chilli: use fresh, ground or as dried chilli (red pepper) flakes; chilli is very hot, so use sparingly. You can always add more heat to a dish, but it's hard to tone down once added. Wash your hands thoroughly after chopping fresh chillies and don't rub your eyes.

Cinnamon: this comes ground or whole in rolled bark sticks. It has a warm, mild and spicy flavour and can be added to curries, rice and desserts.

Coriander: the dried berries of the coriander (cilantro) herb can be used whole in aromatic dishes or ground into a powder.

Cumin: this is used whole as seeds or ground to add warmth to curries and North African dishes.

Curry powder and pastes: these may be mild and spicy or hot, Indian mixes or Thai red and green pastes. Use sparingly, depending on how much heat you like. Check the calorie and fat content, as some pastes have added oil.

Ginger: the fresh root tastes best and can be peeled, then chopped or grated before adding to stir-fries, curries, laksa and other spicy food.

Nutmeg: Buy whole nutmeg and grate it freshly into curries, soups, sauces and desserts.

Paprika: milder than cayenne, paprika may be hot, sweet or even smoked. It is used extensively in Hungarian and Spanish food.

Saffron: saffron strands are expensive, but a little goes a long way and adds a glorious golden colour and subtle flavour to rice, paella and risotto.

Star anise: a star-shaped seed pod with an aniseed flavoured used in Chinese dishes.

Turmeric: this spice is widely used in Indian cooking to flavour curries and colour rice yellow.

# 'Traffic light' foods

The best way to eat yourself thin is to choose foods you enjoy and that fill you up, so you don't feel hungry at the end of a meal. Low-fat, low-calorie vegetables and foods that you have to chew slowly are particularly effective. You can continue to eat most foods as part of a healthy weight-loss or maintenance regime but there are some that are so high in calories, sugar or fat that they are best avoided. Use this helpful 'traffic lights' guide for quick and easy reference.

## Green foods – Go!
Eat these foods freely as part of your daily plan

**Meat:** lean beef, lamb, pork, veal (all visible fat removed), grilled or roasted with spray oil; liver, kidneys
**Cooked meats:** ham, gammon (all visible fat removed)
**Poultry:** chicken, turkey (skin removed), grilled, poached or roasted with spray oil
**Fish and shellfish:** all white fish, grilled, baked or steamed; fresh tuna or canned in spring water; squid (grilled, not fried), mussels, clams, oysters, scallops, prawns (shrimp), white crabmeat, lobster
**Eggs:** not fried
**Dairy:** skimmed (lowfat) milk (cow's, goat's or soy), 0% fat Greek yogurt, very low-fat plain yogurt
**Cheese:** low-fat cottage cheese, Quark, virtually fat-free fromage frais
**Dressings and sauces:** oil-free vinaigrette and dressings, extra-light mayonnaise, soy sauce, nam pla (Thai fish sauce), mustard, vinegars, low-fat stock cubes
**Pasta and noodles:** all plain varieties (not filled pasta) boiled, in small quantities
**Rice:** brown, basmati, Thai fragrant, boiled or steamed, in small quantities
**Whole grains:** bulgur wheat, quinoa, couscous (in small quantities)
**Oats:** oatmeal, porridge (rolled) oats, unsweetened muesli
**Breakfast cereals:** Weetabix, Shredded Wheat (not filled)
**Nuts:** chestnuts
**Pulses:** lentils (Puy, green, brown, red and yellow split); dried beans (black, borlotti, butter/lima, cannellini, chickpeas, haricot, kidney, soya/edamame) or canned
**Vegetarian foods:** Quorn, tofu
**Vegetables:** green leafy vegetables, broccoli, cauliflower, green beans, mushrooms, (bell) peppers, aubergine (eggplant), courgette (zucchini), pumpkin, onions, leeks, celery, fennel, carrots, swede (rutabaga), chillies
**Salads:** all salad leaves, cucumber, radishes, tomatoes, spring onions (scallions)
**Herbs and spices:** all dried and fresh herbs and spices
**Fruit:** apples, pears, peaches, nectarines, oranges, clementines, satsumas, lemons, limes, grapefruit, apricots, plums, pineapple, cherries, strawberries, raspberries, blueberries, cranberries, redcurrants, kiwi fruit, papaya, melon, pomegranate
**Bakery:** high-fibre crispbreads and crackers with less than 5% fat; rice cakes
**Snacks and sweets:** no-sugar jelly (jello)
**Spreads:** Marmite, yeast extract
**Drinks:** Water, tea and coffee (with skimmed/lowfat milk), herbal tea, zero-calorie soft drinks

# Amber foods – Caution!
Go carefully and eat these foods in moderation

**Meat:** minced (ground) beef, lamb and pork (less than 5% fat), low-fat sausages, very lean back (Canadian) bacon (all visible fat removed); beef burgers

**Cured meats:** Parma (prosciutto) and Serrano ham (all visible fat removed)

**Poultry:** duck

**Fish and shellfish:** salmon, herring, mackerel, sardines, grilled, baked or poached, no more than twice weekly; smoked salmon

**Dairy:** semi-skimmed (half fat) milk (cow's, goat's or soy); low-fat spread; low-fat ice cream

**Cheese:** reduced-fat Cheddar, low-fat mozzarella and feta; light soft cheese, grated Parmesan on pasta (no more than 1 teaspoon)

**Dressings and sauces:** sweet chilli sauce, light mayonnaise, reduced-fat tomato salsa, mango chutney, tomato ketchup, horseradish sauce, low-fat custard, miso

**Pasta and noodles:** gnocchi, filled pasta (tortelloni, ravioli, etc.)

**Rice:** risotto, paella, biryani

**Oats:** oatcakes, sweetened muesli

**Breakfast cereals:** granola, cereal bars with less than 5% fat and low sugar content

**Nuts:** peanuts, cashews, pecans, walnuts, Brazil nuts, hazelnuts, pistachios, almonds, pine nuts, coconut, reduced-fat coconut milk

**Seeds:** pumpkin, sesame, sunflower

**Vegetables:** starchy vegetables such as potatoes, parsnips, sweet potatoes, yams, plantains, boiled, baked or dry-roasted; sweetcorn; peas (fresh or frozen); broad beans; olives

**Salads:** beetroot, low-fat coleslaw

**Fruit:** banana, mango, grapes, avocado, dried fruits

**Pastry:** filo (brushed with egg, not butter or oil)

**Bakery:** wholemeal and multigrain bread, tortillas, wraps, pittas, chapatis (check fat grams and calories)

**Desserts and sweets**: meringues, fruit salad in unsweetened natural juice, low-sugar jam (jelly), honey

**Drinks:** fruit juices – drink in moderation; many are high in sugar; fruit smoothies; fruit squash, cordials and flavoured drinks; alcohol (light beer, wine, spirits) – mix spirits with soda water, sparkling mineral water or low-calorie mixers

---

**Low-fat pies and pastry**

Filo pastry (dough) is a healthier alternative to shortcrust and puff pastry. The sheets are so thin and it doesn't contain any fat – only flour and water. You can use it for topping pies as well as for wrapping savoury and fruit mixtures. When layering and assembling the sheets, brush them lightly with some beaten egg or just the egg white rather than oil or melted butter. When you take the sheets out of a packet, always cover them with a damp cloth to prevent them drying out.

---

**Sugar by any other name**

Sugar is often listed under other names on food packaging labels. Look for the following: corn syrup, dextrose, fructose, fruit sugar, glucose, lactose, maltose, molasses and sucrose.

# Red foods – Stop!

Avoid the following or eat occasionally in very small quantities

**Meat:** sausages (with more than 5% fat), spare ribs, belly pork, fatty meat or meat roasted in fat, deep-fried meat
**Cooked meats:** salami, chorizo, pepperoni, pâté
**Poultry:** fried chicken
**Fish and shellfish:** fried fish, deep-fried scampi
**Dairy:** full-fat (whole) milk, cream, soured cream, crème fraîche, butter, ghee; full-fat ice cream; sweetened full-fat (whole) creamy yogurts
**Cheese:** full-fat (whole) and creamy cheeses, e.g. blue cheese, hard cheeses such as Cheddar, Brie, Camembert, cream cheese
**Oils and fats:** sunflower, rapeseed (canola), coconut, vegetable, avocado, grapeseed, corn oils; lard (shortening), dripping; margarine

**Dressings and sauces:** creamy sauces, hollandaise, béarnaise, tartare, mayonnaise, salad cream, salad dressings, e.g. blue cheese, Thousand Island, vinaigrette made with oil, guacamole, full-fat hummus, taramasalata
**Pasta and noodles:** pasta in creamy sauces; fried noodles
**Rice:** fried rice and arancini (rice balls)
**Oats:** porridge (oatmeal) with cream or full-fat (whole) milk and sugar
**Breakfast cereals:** sweetened brands, cereal bars with a high-sugar content and more than 5% fat
**Nuts:** peanut butter and nut spreads; nut brittle; satay sauce; creamed coconut, full-fat (whole) coconut milk
**Vegetables:** fat-roasted, fried or battered vegetables, such as French fries and onion rings

**Fruit:** fruit canned in syrup
Confectionery and spreads: chocolate bars, chocolate spreads, sweets (candy), candied popcorn
**Bakery:** white and brown bread, croissants, brioche, doughnuts, Danish pastries, cakes, muffins; pizza (especially deep pan)
**Pastry:** shortcrust, flaky, puff, hot water crust, choux; pork pies; quiches
**Confectionery and spreads:** potato crisps (chips), tortilla chips, biscuits (cookies), sugar, maple syrup, golden (corn) syrup, molasses, treacle, most desserts, especially cheesecake, pies, tarts
**Drinks:** fortified wines, liqueurs, beer and cider, cocktails, sweetened soft drinks, e.g. cola; latte and cappuccino made with full-fat (whole) milk

# Basic recipes

Here are some basic low-calorie, low-fat recipes that are quick and easy to make and will enhance the flavours of your meals, making them even more delicious.

## Low-fat white sauce

This quantity of white sauce is enough to use in a lasagne or vegetable gratin to feed six people, which works out at 43 calories and a trace of fat per serving. This is a fraction of the calories and fat grams in a regular white sauce made with flour, butter and full-fat (whole) milk.

2 tbsp cornflour (cornstarch)
300ml/½ pint/1¼ cups skimmed (lowfat) milk
100g/3½ oz/scant ½ cup virtually fat-free fromage frais
½ tsp Dijon mustard (optional)
pinch of grated nutmeg
salt and freshly ground black pepper

Blend the cornflour with a little of the milk. Heat the remaining milk in a small non-stick saucepan and bring to the boil.

Reduce the heat and stir in the cornflour mixture with a wooden spoon. Cook over a low heat for 1–2 minutes, stirring all the time, until the sauce thickens and is smooth.

Remove the pan from the heat and beat in the fromage frais, mustard (if using) and nutmeg with a wooden spoon. Season to taste with salt and pepper.

Makes 300ml/½ pint/1¼ cups
Prep and cook: 10 minutes

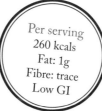

Per serving
260 kcals
Fat: 1g
Fibre: trace
Low GI

## Yogurt salad dressing

This dressing is good for drizzling over sweet cherry tomatoes or some crisp iceberg lettuce and cucumber. Alternatively, use with salad and grilled lamb or chicken in a pitta or wrap. If you use 0% fat Greek yogurt, the calories will be the same but the dressing will be thicker and will be fat-free.

150ml/¼ pint/⅔ cup very low-fat plain yogurt
few fresh mint sprigs, chopped
few fresh coriander (cilantro) sprigs, chopped
good squeeze of lemon juice
salt and freshly ground black pepper

Mix the yogurt, chopped herbs and lemon juice together in a bowl. Season to taste with salt and pepper.

Makes 150ml/¼ pint/⅔ cup
Prep: 5 minutes

Per serving
80 kcals
Fat: 1.5g
Fibre: trace
Low GI

## Asian salad dressing

Use this aromatic dressing to toss a Thai or Vietnamese beef or chicken salad while it's still warm.

juice of 1 lime
1 tsp dark soy sauce
3 tbsp nam pla (Thai fish sauce)
pinch of golden (unrefined) caster (superfine) sugar
1 garlic clove
1 red chilli, deseeded and diced

Mix all the dressing ingredients together in a bowl, stirring until the sugar dissolves.

Makes about 75ml/2½fl oz/⅓ cup
Prep: 5 minutes

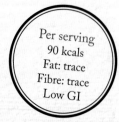

Per serving
90 kcals
Fat: trace
Fibre: trace
Low GI

Variation
Add a little grated fresh ginger without affecting the calorie and fat content.

## Low-fat tomato salsa

Salsa is a great way to flavour Mexican fajitas and quesadillas or as a garnish for a spicy bean soup. You can also serve it as a low-calorie relish with grilled chicken, meat, prawns (shrimp) or roasted vegetables.

3 medium juicy tomatoes, peeled, deseeded and chopped
½ red onion, finely chopped
1 red chilli, deseeded and chopped
few fresh coriander (cilantro) sprigs, chopped
juice of 1 lime
freshly ground black pepper

In a bowl, mix together the tomatoes, onion, chilli, coriander and lime juice. Season with pepper. This salsa will keep for a couple of days in a covered container in the refrigerator.

Makes about 150g/5½oz
Prep: 10 minutes

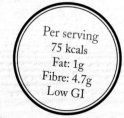

Per serving
75 kcals
Fat: 1g
Fibre: 4.7g
Low GI

Variations
Add crushed roasted garlic cloves or a small red or yellow (bell) pepper, which has been deseeded and diced. This will add 30 kcals, 0.3g fat and 1.6g fibre.

## Pesto fromage frais

Use this as a dip for raw vegetable sticks and cherry tomatoes, or serve as a sauce with grilled chicken, vegetables or fish.
This makes enough to serve four people (25 calories and 0.5g fat per serving).

150g/5½oz/⅔ cup virtually fat-free natural fromage frais
1 tbsp reduced-fat green pesto
salt and freshly ground black pepper
few fresh chives, snipped

In a bowl, mix together the fromage frais and pesto until well blended. Season to taste with salt and pepper and sprinkle with snipped chives.

Makes 150g/5½oz
Prep: 5 minutes

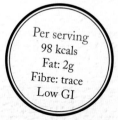

Per serving
98 kcals
Fat: 2g
Fibre: trace
Low GI

## Exotic fruit salsa

This is enough salsa for six servings. The natural sweetness of the mango and papaya complement the fiery chilli.

100g/3½oz mango, diced
100g/3½oz papaya, diced
½ red onion, finely chopped
1 small red (bell) pepper, deseeded and diced
1 hot red chilli, deseeded and finely chopped
juice of 1 lime
salt and freshly ground black pepper
few fresh coriander (cilantro) sprigs,
    chopped

Mix all the ingredients together in a bowl. Cover and chill in the refrigerator until required. This will keep for a couple of days.

Makes about 300g/10½oz
Prep: 15 minutes

Per serving
150 kcals
Fat: 1g
Fibre: 5g
Low GI

Variation
Add 50g/1¾oz quartered baby plum tomatoes. This adds 9 kcals, 0.1g fat and 0.5g fibre to the salsa.

## Tzatziki

This is enough tzatziki to feed six people as a dip or a sauce to serve with grilled fish, chicken, lamb or vegetables. Alternatively, use to top a salad or add to pitta bread fillings.

300g/10½oz/1¼ cups 0% fat Greek yogurt
½ cucumber, peeled and diced
2 garlic cloves, crushed
squeeze of lemon juice
salt and freshly ground black pepper
small bunch of fresh mint, chopped

Mix all the ingredients together in a bowl, then cover and chill in the refrigerator for at least 30 minutes to bring out the flavours.

Makes about 400g/14oz
Prep: 10 minutes

Per serving
170 kcals
Fat: 0.2g
Fibre: 1g
Low GI

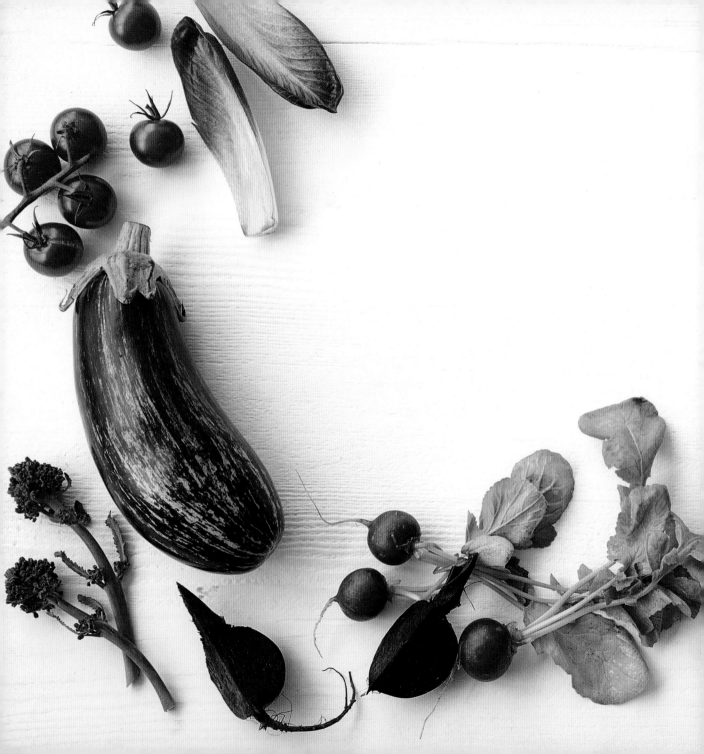

# 100 calories

# HI-FIBRE BREAKFAST MUFFINS

**A great way to start the day – and a real treat. Adding wheat bran to the muffin mixture boosts their fibre content. You can make them in advance, but because they contain fresh fruit, they must be kept in the fridge.**

150ml/¼ pint/⅝ cup skimmed (lowfat) milk
60g/2¼oz wheat bran
60g/2¼oz soft brown sugar
1 large free-range egg
100g/3½oz plain (all-purpose) flour
pinch each of ground cinnamon and grated nutmeg
½ tsp baking powder
½ tsp bicarbonate of soda (baking soda)
125g/4½oz/generous ¾ cup fresh blueberries, cranberries or raspberries

Makes 8 muffins
Prep: 15 minutes
Soak: 10 minutes
Cook: 20 minutes

Preheat the oven to 190°C/375°F/Gas mark 5. Line a muffin tin with eight paper cases.

Put the milk and wheat bran in a bowl and stir well. Leave to soak for 10 minutes.

Beat the sugar and egg together until well combined, then beat in the milk and bran mixture.

Sift in the flour, cinnamon, nutmeg, baking powder and bicarbonate of soda and fold in gently in a figure of eight motion with a metal spoon. Stir in the berries, taking care to distribute them evenly through the mixture.

Divide the mixture between the paper cases and bake for 20 minutes, or until the muffins have risen and are firm to the touch.

Cool the muffins on a wire rack, then store in a sealed container in the refrigerator.

Per muffin
100 kcals
Fat: 1.5g
Fibre: 3.5g
Medium GI

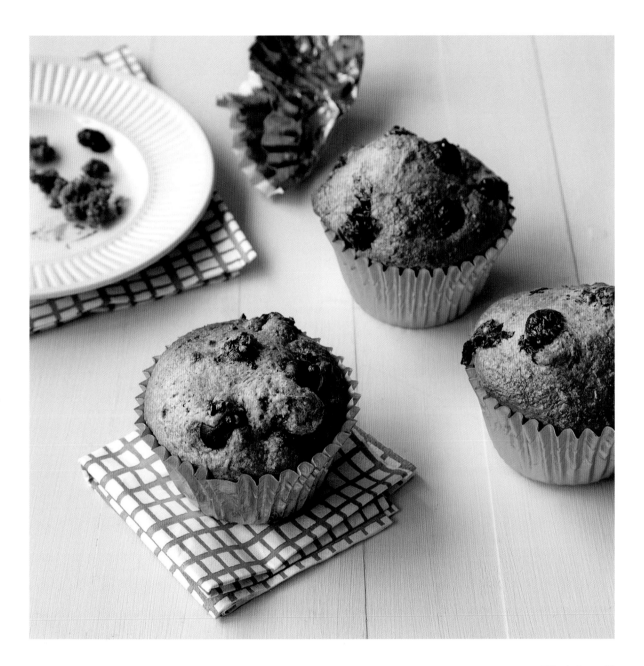

# SCRAMBLED EGG AND SMOKED SALMON MINI BLINIS

**You don't have to use expensive smoked salmon for this recipe – you can buy trimmings in most supermarkets at half the price. Although it's relatively high in calories and fat, it's so strongly flavoured that a little goes a long way. These blinis are perfect for serving as party canapés, too.**

4 cocktail blinis
1 large free-range egg
1 tsp water
freshly ground black pepper
40g/1½oz smoked salmon, chopped
few fresh chives, snipped

Serves 2
Prep: 5 minutes
Cook: 2 minutes

Preheat the oven to 190°C/375°F/Gas mark 5.

Place the cocktail blinis on a baking sheet and pop into the oven for a few minutes, or according to the packet instructions.

Break the egg into a small bowl and add the water and some pepper. Beat with a fork or whisk until the white and yolk are combined.

Heat a small non-stick saucepan over a low heat and pour the beaten egg into the hot pan. Stir gently with a wooden spoon and, as soon as the egg starts to scramble, stir in the smoked salmon and chives.

Divide the scrambled egg mixture between the warm blinis and serve immediately.

Per serving
100 kcals
Fat: 5g
Fibre: trace
Medium GI

# KICKSTART BANANA BERRY SMOOTHIE

**Breakfast in a glass – quick and simple to make, very healthy and practically no washing-up. A lot of people think that all smoothies are low in calories, but they're not, especially if large bananas (double the calories of small ones), full-fat milk, creamy yogurt or coconut milk are added; always check the ingredients carefully.**

1 juicy peach
1 small banana, peeled
100g/3½oz/generous ⅔ cup strawberries, hulled
100g/3½oz/scant ½ cup very low-fat plain yogurt
1 tsp linseeds (flaxseeds)

Serves 2
Prep: 5 minutes

Cut the peach in half and remove the stone, then cut the flesh into chunks.

Place the peach, banana, strawberries, yogurt and linseeds in a blender or food processor. With the top of the blender held firmly in place, blitz until everything is well combined and smooth. If the smoothie is too thick for your taste, you can add a little water to get the desired consistency.

Pour the smoothie into two glasses and serve. Alternatively, transfer the smoothie to a jug and chill in the refrigerator for an hour or so, but not too long because the banana will discolour after a while.

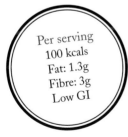

Per serving
100 kcals
Fat: 1.3g
Fibre: 3g
Low GI

OR TRY THIS…
INSTEAD OF USING A PEACH, SUBSTITUTE A RIPE
NECTARINE OR 50G/1¾OZ PEELED RIPE MANGO.
OR USE RASPBERRIES INSTEAD OF STRAWBERRIES.

# SPICED SWEET POTATO WEDGES

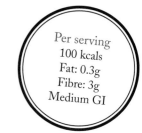

Per serving
100 kcals
Fat: 0.3g
Fibre: 3g
Medium GI

**These spicy wedges dipped into a fresh mango salsa taste so good that it's hard to believe that one portion is only 100 calories – after all, a 50g/2oz bag of potato crisps (chips) has approximately 250 calories and they don't fill you up. This is another great idea for parties. And you can use the salsa with grilled chicken, steak or pork.**

1 x 125g/4½oz sweet potato, unpeeled, washed or scrubbed and cut into wedges
spray olive oil
pinch each of ground coriander, cumin and chilli powder
sea salt and freshly ground black pepper
1 tbsp chopped fresh coriander (cilantro)

**For the mango salsa**
100g/3½oz ripe mango, peeled and diced
1 ripe tomato, chopped
1 spring onion (scallion), finely chopped
¼ yellow (bell) pepper, deseeded and chopped
½ small red chilli, deseeded and chopped
salt and freshly ground black pepper
juice of ½ lime
1 tbsp chopped fresh coriander (cilantro) leaves

Serves 2
Prep: 5 minutes
Cook: 15–20 minutes

Preheat the oven to 200°C/400°F/Gas mark 6.

Spray the sweet potato wedges lightly with oil, then coat them with the ground spices. Place them on a non-stick baking sheet and bake for 15–20 minutes until the sweet potato is tender and crisp and golden on the outside.

Meanwhile, mix all the ingredients for the salsa in a small bowl.

Sprinkle the cooked wedges with a little sea salt and a grinding of pepper. Sprinkle with coriander and serve immediately with the mango salsa dip.

OR TRY THIS...
USE A BAKING POTATO INSTEAD OF THE SWEET POTATO AND YOU WILL SAVE ABOUT 10 CALORIES PER SERVING. SCRUB THE POTATO, CUT INTO WEDGES AND SPICE IN THE SAME WAY. BAKE IN THE PREHEATED OVEN FOR 40–50 MINUTES, UNTIL TENDER INSIDE AND GOLDEN BROWN AND CRISP ON THE OUTSIDE.

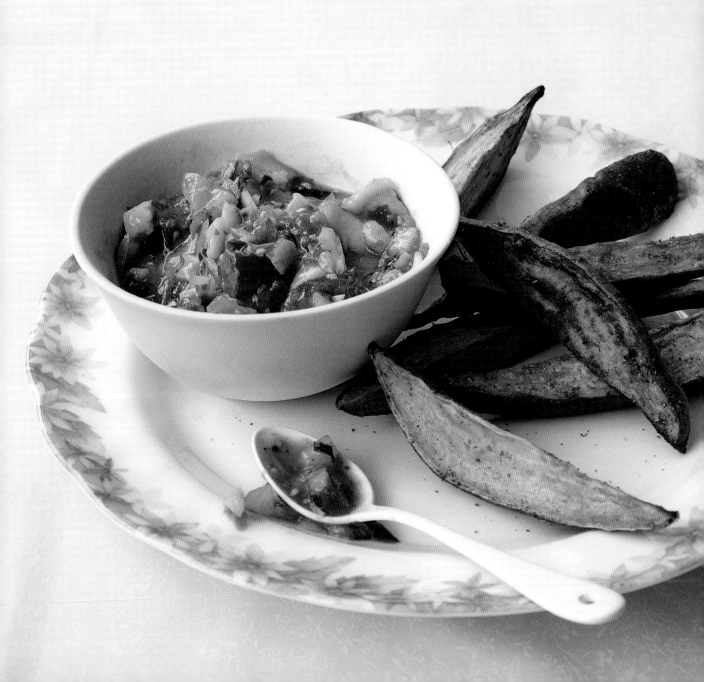

# ROSEMARY-SKEWERED VEGETABLES

**It's fun to use fresh rosemary stems as skewers for vegetables, chicken and meat. They look great and they impart a subtle flavour to the food. You will need strong, woody stems. Strip most of the leaves off first, just leaving the ones on the end intact.**

6 sturdy fresh rosemary stems

½ red (bell) pepper, deseeded and cut into chunks

½ yellow (bell) pepper, deseeded and cut into chunks

1 courgette (zucchini), cut into chunks

1 small red onion, cut into chunks

2 fresh thyme sprigs, leaves picked

salt and freshly ground black pepper

spray olive oil

**For the creamy pesto dip**

85g/3oz/generous ⅓ cup virtually fat-free fromage frais

2 tsp reduced-fat green pesto

20 fresh basil leaves, chopped

1 ripe tomato, peeled and chopped

dash of lemon juice

Serves 2
Prep: 15 minutes
Cook: 10 minutes

To make the dip, mix the fromage frais with the pesto and basil leaves. Stir in the chopped tomato and lemon juice and season to taste with freshly ground black pepper. Cover and chill in the refrigerator until required.

Preheat the grill (broiler). Strip off most of the leaves from the rosemary stems, just leaving a few on the tip of each one.

Thread the pepper chunks onto the rosemary skewers, alternating with the chunks of courgette and red onion.

Put the kebabs on a foil-lined grill pan and sprinkle with the thyme leaves, then season with salt and pepper. Spray lightly with oil. Cook under the hot grill, turning occasionally, until the vegetables are just tender and slightly charred on the edges.

Serve the warm kebabs with the pesto dip.

Per serving
100 kcals
Fat: 4.5g
Fibre: 0.7g
Medium GI

OR TRY THIS...
USE REDUCED-FAT RED PESTO INSTEAD OF GREEN –
THE CALORIES WILL BE APPROXIMATELY THE SAME.

# PESTO VEGGIE MINI TARTLETS

Per serving
100 kcals
Fat: 3g
Fibre: 1.5g
Medium GI

**If you brush the filo pastry with just the beaten egg white and omit the yolk, you will reduce the calories and fat content even more. These tartlets are very colourful and are perfect for entertaining.**

spray olive oil
¼ small red onion, finely chopped
1 small courgette (zucchini), diced
1 small red or yellow (bell) pepper, deseeded and diced
4 cherry tomatoes, chopped
few drops of balsamic vinegar
freshly ground black pepper
2 x 15g/½oz sheets filo pastry (dough)
2 tsp beaten egg, for brushing
1 tsp reduced-fat green pesto
30g/1oz reduced-fat mozzarella, diced

Serves 2
Prep: 15 minutes
Cook: 20–25 minutes

Preheat the oven to 190°C/375°F/Gas mark 5.

Lightly spray a frying pan with oil and place over a low heat. Add the onion, courgette and pepper and cook for about 5 minutes, stirring occasionally, until tender.

Stir in the tomatoes and cook for 2–3 minutes. Season with balsamic vinegar and pepper, then remove from the heat.

Lightly spray four small tartlet tins with oil. Cut each sheet of filo pastry into six squares and brush each one lightly with beaten egg. Layer them up, three squares in each tin, with the edges overlapping the sides slightly.

Brush the pesto lightly over the inside of each tartlet, then fill the pastry cases with the vegetables and scatter the mozzarella over the top.

Bake the tartlets in the oven for 12–15 minutes, or until the mozzarella has melted and the filo pastry is crisp and golden. Serve hot or warm.

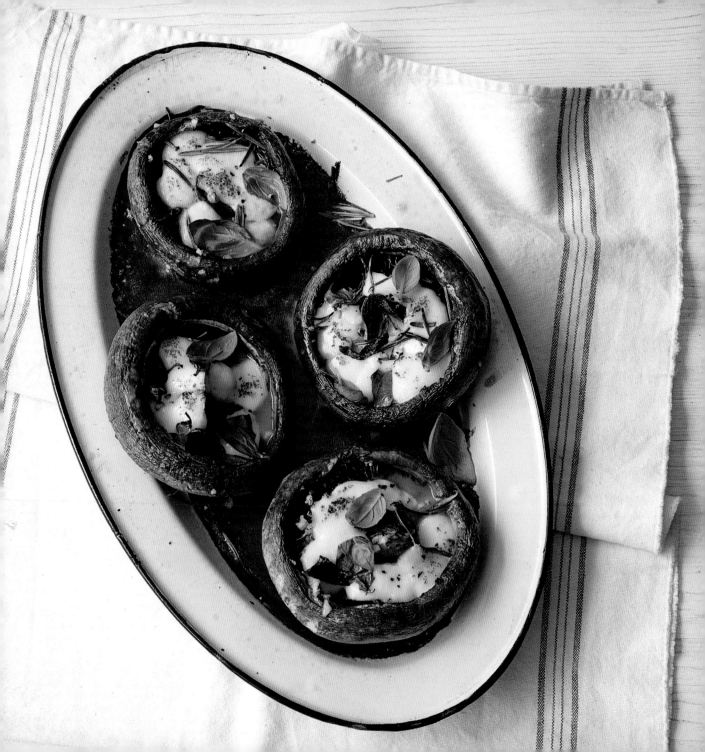

# ITALIAN PORTOBELLO MUSHROOM MELTS

Large mushrooms are extremely versatile low-fat food. They can be used as a base for vegetable stacks or 'pizzas', or they can be filled with low-calorie stuffings and fillings. They have a 'meaty' texture, which is very satisfying and filling. If you don't have any passata (available in jars and packets in most supermarkets), you can use canned chopped tomato instead for a more chunky result.

150g/5½oz passata (strained tomatoes)
4 large Portobello or field mushrooms
2 garlic cloves, crushed
spray olive oil
85g/3oz reduced-fat mozzarella cheese, diced
2 fresh rosemary sprigs, leaves picked
2 fresh basil sprigs, chopped, plus extra leaves to serve
salt and freshly ground black pepper

Serves 2
Prep: 10 minutes
Cook: 15 minutes

Per serving
100 kcals
Fat: 5g
Fibre: 1g
Low GI

Preheat the oven to 190°C/375°F/Gas mark 5.

Pour the passata into a shallow ovenproof dish and arrange the mushrooms on top, stalk-side up. Sprinkle the garlic into the mushrooms and spray lightly with oil. Scatter the mozzarella and herbs over the top and season with salt and pepper.

Bake in the oven for 15 minutes, or until the mushrooms are cooked and tender, and the mozzarella has melted and is golden brown. Serve immediately, scattered with basil leaves.

OR TRY THIS...
ADD A LITTLE DICED COURGETTE (ZUCCHINI), (BELL) PEPPER OR AUBERGINE (EGGPLANT) TO THE PASSATA.

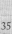

# LEBANESE STUFFED PEPPER ROLLS

**These colourful roll-ups can be wrapped in clingfilm (plastic wrap) and taken to work as a packed lunch – much more diet-friendly than sandwiches and regular wraps. As a finishing touch, try drizzling a few drops of balsamic vinegar over them.**

2 x 100g/3½oz yellow (bell) peppers
30g/1oz/scant ¼ cup bulgur wheat
1 juicy tomato, deseeded and chopped
¼ red onion, finely chopped
2 tbsp chopped fresh flat-leaf parsley
2 tbsp chopped fresh mint
2 black olives, pitted and chopped
salt and freshly ground black pepper
juice of 1 lemon

Prep: 15 minutes
Soak: 15 minutes
Chill: 30 minutes
Cook: 4–5 minutes

Preheat the grill (broiler). Place the peppers under the hot grill, turning occasionally, until the skins are blistered and start to char. Pop them into a plastic bag and leave until they are cool enough to handle, then peel off the skins and cut them in half. Discard the cores and seeds, then trim the pepper halves so that you end up with eight rectangles. Dice the trimmings and set aside.

Put the bulgur wheat in a bowl and cover with cold water. Leave to soak for 15 minutes, then rinse and drain well, squeezing out any excess water.

Mix the bulgur with the chopped tomato, onion, parsley, mint, black olives and the reserved diced yellow pepper. Season to taste with salt and pepper, then stir in the lemon juice.

Divide the mixture between the pepper rectangles and then roll them up like Swiss rolls (jelly rolls). Wrap in clingfilm and chill in the refrigerator for at least 30 minutes before eating.

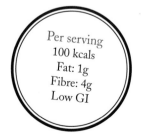

Per serving
100 kcals
Fat: 1g
Fibre: 4g
Low GI

# CHICKPEA MASH AND VEGGIE DIPPERS

**You can use this chickpea mash to accompany grilled fish, lamb or chicken, or as a 'dip' for vegetables. Don't over-blend the chickpeas – they should have a coarse texture rather than being too smooth. If you like spicy flavours, add some finely chopped chilli or a good pinch of ground cumin. Or serve it with a dash of fiery red harissa paste.**

250g/9oz mixed baby green vegetables, such as asparagus tips, courgettes (zucchini), fine green beans, tenderstem broccoli
125g/4½oz canned chickpeas, drained
1 garlic clove, crushed
good pinch of smoked sweet paprika, plus extra for sprinkling
juice of ½ small lemon
salt and freshly ground black pepper

Serves 2
Prep: 10 minutes
Cook: 8–12 minutes

Set a saucepan of water over a high heat and bring to the boil. Add the vegetables in batches and cook for 2–3 minutes until just tender but they still retain their 'bite'. Remove with a slotted spoon and plunge them into a bowl of iced water.

Put the chickpeas in a blender or food processor with the garlic, paprika and lemon juice. Blitz to a coarse paste, then season to taste with salt and pepper. If it's too thick, you can thin it with a little water (save the blanching water from the vegetables, if wished) or some more lemon juice.

When the vegetables are cool, remove them from the iced water and drain well. Pat them dry with kitchen paper.

Sprinkle the chickpea mash with a dusting of paprika and serve with the vegetables.

Per serving
100 kcals
Fat: 1.8g
Fibre: 6g
Low GI

# MEDITERRANEAN NO-PASTRY QUICHES

**What makes quiche so high in calories is the pastry case in which it is usually made. By getting rid of the pastry, the quiches are more like muffins and can be eaten for breakfast, or as a snack or packed lunch. You can vary the vegetable fillings, adding chopped spinach, sautéed leek, mushrooms and courgette (zucchini), depending on your personal taste.**

spray olive oil
½ small red onion, finely chopped
½ small yellow (bell) pepper, deseeded and finely chopped
1 ripe tomato, chopped
1 free-range medium egg
2 tbsp skimmed (lowfat) milk
few fresh chives, snipped
50g/1¾oz/scant ¼ cup low-fat cottage cheese
salt and freshly ground black pepper

Makes 2
Prep: 10 minutes
Cook: 25–30 minutes

Preheat the oven to 190°C/375°F/Gas mark 5.

Lightly spray a frying pan with oil and place over a medium heat. When it's hot, add the onion and yellow pepper and cook for 5 minutes, or until they start to soften. Stir in the tomato and cook for 2 minutes, then remove from the heat.

Lightly spray two deep non-stick muffin tins with oil, or line with baking parchment, and spoon the vegetable mixture into them.

Whisk the egg and milk together. Stir in the chives and cottage cheese, and season with a little salt and pepper.

Pour the beaten egg mixture over the vegetables in the muffin tins, then bake for 20 minutes, or until the quiches are well risen, golden brown and firm to the touch.

You can serve the quiches immediately or leave them to cool and then store in a container in the refrigerator for breakfast or a packed lunch.

Per serving
100 kcals
Fat: 4g
Fibre: 1.5g
Low GI

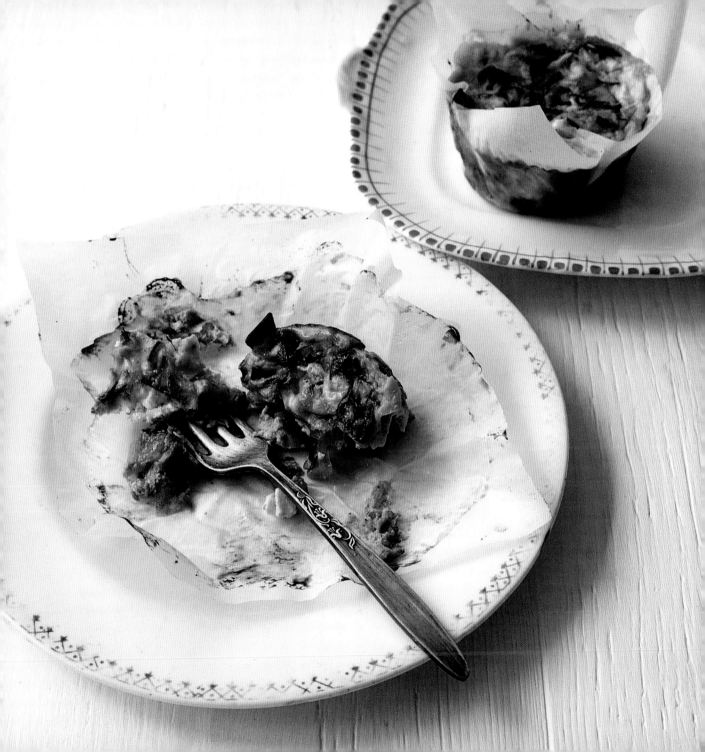

# INDONESIAN CHICKEN SATAY

**If you use bamboo skewers, soak them in a bowl of water for a few minutes before threading the chicken onto them. This will prevent them burning during cooking. You can substitute turkey breast for chicken and the calories and fat grams will stay the same. Serve with cucumber strips, if wished.**

100g/3½oz boneless, skinless chicken breasts
juice of 1 lime
1 garlic clove, crushed
1 tbsp ground coriander
1 tbsp ground cumin
½ tsp turmeric

**For the satay dip**
50ml/1¾fl oz/scant ¼ cup canned reduced-fat coconut milk
½ tsp curry paste
10g/⅓oz reduced-fat peanut butter
squeeze of lemon juice

Serves 2
Prep: 10 minutes
Chill: 1 hour
Cook: 10 minutes

Place the chicken breasts between two sheets of clingfilm (plastic wrap) and beat with a rolling pin until thin. Cut each breast into three long strips, about 2.5cm/1in wide and place in a shallow dish.

Mix the lime juice, garlic and spices to a paste and spoon over the chicken. Stir well, then cover and marinate in the refrigerator for at least 1 hour.

Meanwhile, make the satay dip: heat the coconut milk and curry paste in a small saucepan over a low heat for 3–4 minutes, stirring. Stir in the peanut butter and lemon juice, and heat through, stirring. Remove from the heat and leave to cool.

Preheat the grill (broiler). Remove the chicken from the spicy marinade and thread each piece onto a thin bamboo skewer. Place them in a foil-lined grill pan.

Cook under the hot grill for about 10 minutes, turning occasionally, until the chicken is slightly charred and golden brown on the outside, and thoroughly cooked inside.

Serve the hot kebabs with the satay sauce for dipping.

Per serving
100 kcals
Fat: 4.5g
Fibre: 0.7g
Low GI

# SPICED BUFFALO WINGS

Aromatic sticky chicken wings are delicious finger food, but you must remember to remove the skin from the wings before marinating them to reduce the fat content. Virtually fat-free fromage frais is the slimmer's friend; it can be flavoured with herbs, spices, grated lemon or lime zest, finely chopped spring onions (scallions) or a drizzle of sweet chilli sauce to make low-calorie dips and sauces.

1 tsp hoisin sauce
1 tsp tomato ketchup
2 tsp dark soy sauce
½ tsp sweet chilli sauce
1 garlic clove, crushed
grated zest and juice of ½ orange
3 x 85g/3oz chicken wings, skinned and cut in half

**For the honey mustard dip**
50g/1¾oz/scant ¼ cup virtually fat-free natural fromage frais
1 tsp honey mustard
few fresh chives, snipped

Serves 2
Prep: 10 minutes
Chill: 30 minutes
Cook: 12–15 minutes

Make the honey mustard dip: mix the fromage frais with the mustard in a small bowl and sprinkle the chives over the top. Cover and leave to chill in the refrigerator.

Mix the hoisin sauce, ketchup, soy and chilli sauces, garlic, orange zest and juice together in a bowl.

Add the halved chicken wings and turn them in the hoisin sauce mixture until coated. Cover with clingfilm (plastic wrap) and chill in the refrigerator for at least 30 minutes.

Preheat the grill (broiler). Remove the chicken wings from the marinade and place them on a foil-lined grill pan. Spoon any remaining marinade over the top, then cook under the hot grill for 12–15 minutes, turning occasionally and basting with the marinade.

Serve the hot chicken wings with the honey mustard dip.

Per serving
100 kcals
Fat: 2.5g
Fibre: trace
Low GI

# GRILLED CALIFORNIAN SHRIMP SALAD

**Barbecued and grilled salads are a speciality of some Californian restaurants. The vegetables are cooked very quickly until tender but still al dente (with a bit of bite), tossed in a tangy dressing and eaten warm. If you use green (bell) pepper instead of red or yellow, which are sweeter, you will save about 13 calories per serving.**

125g/4½oz thin asparagus spears, trimmed
½ red (bell) pepper, deseeded and cut into strips
½ yellow (bell) pepper, deseeded and cut into strips
2 spring onions (scallions), trimmed
spray olive oil
1 small radicchio or chicory, trimmed and cut into wedges
150g/5½oz raw tiger prawns (jumbo shrimp), peeled
handful of baby spinach leaves
salt and freshly ground black pepper

**For the dressing**
1 tbsp oil-free vinaigrette
1 tbsp light soy sauce
juice of ½ lemon or lime

Serves 2
Prep: 10 minutes
Cook: 6 minutes

Preheat a barbecue or a ridged griddle pan on top of the stove. Lightly spray the asparagus, peppers and spring onions with oil and place on the barbecue over hot coals or on the hot griddle pan and cook quickly, turning frequently, for 2–3 minutes.

Spray the radicchio lightly with oil and place on the grill with the prawns. Cook for 2 minutes on each side, or until the prawns turn pink. Toss the spinach leaves onto the grill for a few seconds – just long enough to warm and wilt them.

Blend the dressing ingredients together in a small bowl until they emulsify, or shake them in a screwtop jar. Toss the slightly charred barbecued salad vegetables and prawns with the dressing in a serving dish. Season to taste and serve immediately before the salad gets cold.

Per serving
100 kcals
Fat: 1g
Fibre: 3.5g
Low GI

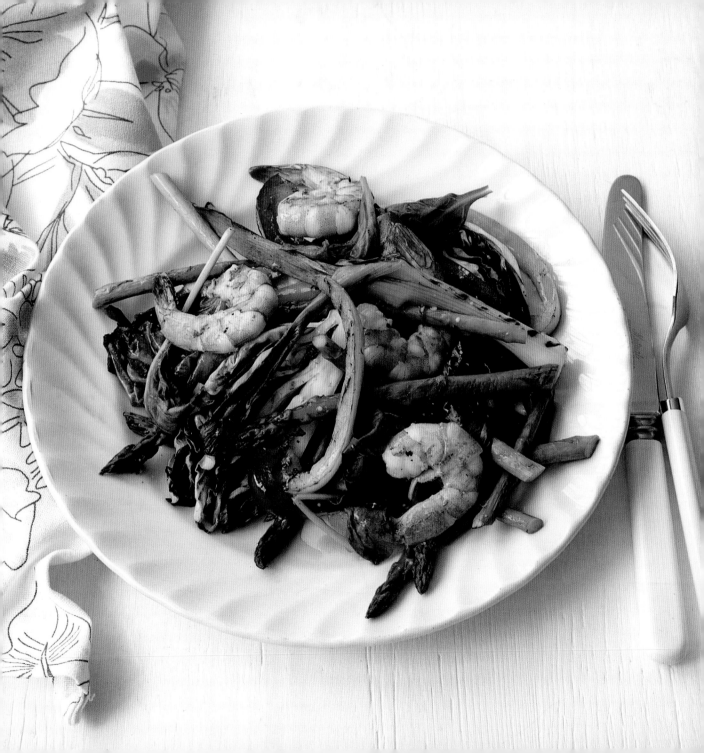

# BAKED CHEESY STUFFED SQUASH

**This makes a filling lunch if you serve the squash with some salad leaves, cucumber and radishes tossed in oil-free dressing. The additional calories will be negligible. Other vegetables, including tomatoes, hollowed-out courgettes (zucchini) and peppers can be stuffed and baked in the same way.**

2 x 100g/3½oz small butternut squashes, halved lengthways and deseeded

spray olive oil

salt and freshly ground black pepper

60g/2¼oz/¼ cup low-fat ricotta cheese

2 spring onions (scallions), chopped

100g/3½oz juicy plum tomatoes, chopped

2 tbsp chopped fresh basil or parsley

Serves 2
Prep: 15 minutes
Cook: 15–20 minutes

Preheat the oven to 190°C/375°F/Gas mark 5.

Put the four butternut squash halves on a baking sheet, hollow-side up. Spray them lightly with oil and season with a little salt and pepper. Bake for 15–20 minutes, or until softened.

Scoop out most of the cooked flesh and chop it roughly. Mix with the ricotta, spring onions, tomatoes and herbs. Spoon the ricotta stuffing back into the hollowed-out shells and serve immediately.

Per serving
100 kcals
Fat: 2.5g
Fibre: 4g
Low GI

OR TRY THIS...
IF YOU CAN'T FIND ANY SMALL SQUASHES, YOU CAN HALVE AND DRESS A 200G/7OZ ONE AND THEN BAKE AND STUFF IT IN THE SAME WAY. EACH HALF WILL BE A SINGLE PORTION. COOK FOR 20 MINUTES.

# SPICED TOFU AND VEGGIE SKEWERS

**Versatile and healthy and beloved of vegetarians, tofu (sometimes known as bean curd) is very low in fat but an excellent source of protein. Because it has a very mild taste, it is often cooked with strongly flavoured herbs and spices or served with hot sauces.**

100g/3½oz butternut squash, peeled and cubed
1 red onion, cut into 8 pieces
spray olive oil
3 fresh thyme sprigs, leaves picked
salt and freshly ground black pepper
150g/5½oz tofu, cubed
85g/3oz wild rocket (arugula)
few drops of balsamic vinegar
2 tsp sweet chilli sauce, to serve

Serves 2
Prep: 15 minutes
Cook: 40–45 minutes

Preheat the oven to 180°C/350°F/Gas mark 4.

Arrange the butternut squash and onion on a baking sheet and spray lightly with oil. Sprinkle with thyme leaves and season with a little salt and pepper. Roast in the oven, turning once or twice, for 30–35 minutes, or until tender.

Spray a frying pan lightly with oil and place over a medium heat. When it's hot, add the tofu cubes and cook for 5 minutes, stirring and turning them occasionally.

Thread the tofu, squash and onion onto skewers and serve with the rocket drizzled with balsamic vinegar, and with a teaspoon of chilli sauce on the side.

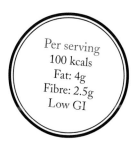

Per serving
100 kcals
Fat: 4g
Fibre: 2.5g
Low GI

# SPANISH ROASTED VEGETABLE SALAD

**In Spain, warm roasted vegetables are often sprinkled with sherry vinegar and crushed garlic – raw or roasted – is added to the dressing. Don't be tempted to mop up the delicious juices with some crusty bread: an average 60g/2¼oz serving packs a hefty 144 calories and 1g fat.**

1 small aubergine (eggplant)
½ red (bell) pepper
½ yellow (bell) pepper
1 Spanish onion, unpeeled
1 courgette (zucchini)
2 ripe tomatoes
2 garlic cloves, unpeeled
spray olive oil
1 tsp red wine vinegar or sherry vinegar
juice of ½ lemon
sea salt and freshly ground black pepper
2 tbsp chopped fresh parsley

Serves 2
Prep: 15 minutes
Cook: 30 minutes

Preheat the oven to 180°C/350°F/Gas mark 4.

Put the aubergine, peppers, onion, courgette and tomatoes in a roasting tin. Tuck the garlic cloves in between them and spray lightly with oil. Roast for 30 minutes, turning them occasionally, or until they are tender and slightly charred.

Cut the aubergine into strips. Peel the peppers, deseed and cut the flesh into strips. Peel the onion and cut into wedges. Slice the courgette thinly, then put all the prepared vegetables in a serving dish.

Peel the tomatoes and garlic cloves and mash them with the vinegar and lemon juice in a small bowl. Toss with the roasted vegetables and season to taste with salt and pepper.

Sprinkle the chopped parsley over the top and leave to cool a little before serving at room temperature – do not chill.

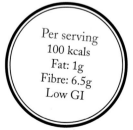

Per serving
100 kcals
Fat: 1g
Fibre: 6.5g
Low GI

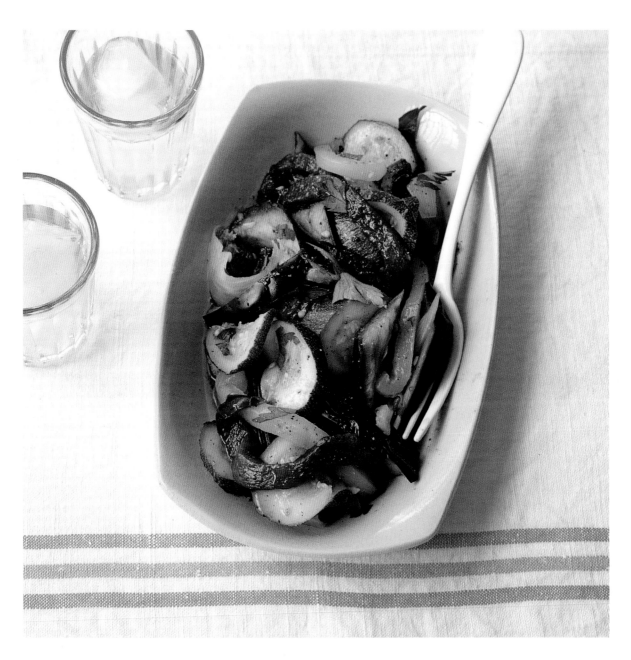

# SPICY WINTER COLESLAW

**Most people buy tubs of coleslaw in the supermarket and never check the labels to read the calorie and fat content. This is a big mistake because 100g/3½oz coleslaw can contain as many as 325 calories and 33g fat (with added cheese) or as little as 60 calories and 2g fat (fat-reduced brands). However, none of them taste as good or as crunchy as this spicy version, which is sweetened with fresh mango.**

85g/3oz white cabbage, finely shredded
85g/3oz red cabbage, finely shredded
1 large carrot, grated
¼ onion, finely grated
85g/3oz diced ripe mango
spray oil
1 tsp black mustard seeds
½ tsp cumin seeds
1 small fresh red chilli, deseeded and finely chopped
1 tsp grated fresh root ginger
125g/4½ oz/½ cup 0% fat Greek yogurt
1 tbsp extra light mayonnaise
juice of 1 small lemon
2 tbsp chopped fresh parsley
salt and freshly ground black pepper

Serves 2
Prep: 15 minutes
Cook: 1 minute

Put the shredded cabbage, grated carrot and onion in a large bowl with the mango.

Lightly spray a small frying pan with oil and place over a high heat. When it's very hot, tip in the mustard and cumin seeds and stir-fry for about 30 seconds, just long enough to release their aroma. Stir in the chilli and ginger, cook for 30 seconds and then remove from the heat.

Mix the spices with the yogurt, mayonnaise and lemon juice. Spoon over the prepared vegetables and mango and toss lightly together until everything is well coated.

Stir in the parsley and season to taste with salt and pepper. Eat immediately or cover and keep in the refrigerator.

Per serving
100 kcals
Fat: 0.8g
Fibre: 5g
Low GI

# MYKONOS HORIATIKI SALAD

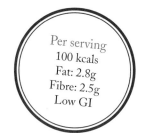

Per serving
100 kcals
Fat: 2.8g
Fibre: 2.5g
Low GI

In every seaside tavern and high-end restaurant all over Greece, horiatiki appears on the menu. The classic Greek salad of juicy tomatoes, cucumber chunks, red onion, peppers and olives, flavoured with oregano and topped with a slice of salty feta cheese, makes a filling light meal. In Greece it is dressed at the table with fruity olive oil and wine vinegar. It's important to use really ripe, full-flavoured tomatoes to get the best and most authentic results.

4 juicy red tomatoes, cut into large chunks
¼ cucumber, cut into large chunks
½ red onion, thinly sliced
1 small green (bell) pepper, halved, deseeded and cut into chunks
6 small black olives
2 tbsp oil-free vinaigrette dressing
juice of ½ lemon
30g/1oz slice of reduced-fat feta cheese
good pinch of dried oregano
freshly ground black pepper

Serves 2
Prep: 10 minutes

Put the tomatoes, cucumber and onion in a salad bowl with the green pepper. Add the olives and mix together lightly.

Whisk the vinaigrette dressing and lemon juice together in a small bowl until well combined, or shake together in a screwtop jar. Pour over the salad and toss lightly.

Place the feta on top of the salad and sprinkle with oregano. Grind a little black pepper over the top and serve immediately. At the table, break up the feta with a fork.

OR TRY THIS…
ADD CHOPPED FRESH HERBS, SUCH AS PARSLEY, MINT AND OREGANO, AT NO EXTRA CALORIES. IF YOU USE A RED OR YELLOW PEPPER INSTEAD OF A GREEN ONE, YOU WILL ADD 10 CALORIES TO EACH SERVING.

# SPICED SQUASH AND BUTTER BEAN SOUP

**A quick and easy soup, which is very substantial and fills you up. If you don't have any canned butter beans, you can use haricot or cannellini instead. The result will taste equally good and the calories will stay the same.**

spray oil
1 onion, chopped
1 garlic clove, crushed
1 fresh red chilli, deseeded and diced
400g/14oz butternut squash, peeled,
deseeded and cubed
900ml/1½ pints/3½ cups vegetable stock
200g/7oz canned butter (lima) beans,
rinsed and drained
pinch each of ground nutmeg,
turmeric and cumin
salt and freshly ground black pepper
4 tsp low-fat plain yogurt
2 tbsp chopped fresh parsley

Serves 4
Prep: 10 minutes
Cook: 35 minutes

Spray a large saucepan lightly with oil and place over a low heat. Add the onion, garlic and chilli and cook for about 5 minutes until the onion starts to soften. Add the squash and cook for about 5 minutes, stirring occasionally.

Add the vegetable stock and bring to the boil. Reduce the heat to a simmer and cook gently for 15 minutes, or until the squash is cooked and tender.

Add half the butter beans to the soup, then blitz the soup in a blender or food processor until smooth.

Pour the soup into a clean pan and stir in the spices and remaining butter beans. Season to taste with salt and pepper and heat through gently.

Serve the hot soup in bowls, topped with a swirl of yogurt and sprinkled with parsley.

Per serving
100 kcals
Fat: 0.5g
Fibre: 3.5g
Low GI

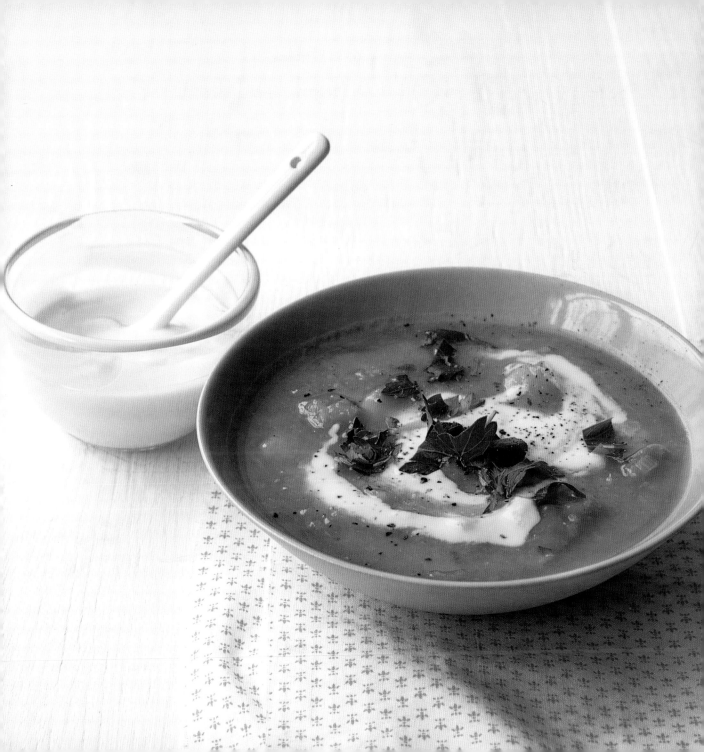

# SPRING GREEN PRAWN PARCELS

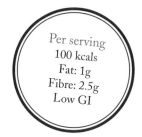
Per serving
100 kcals
Fat: 1g
Fibre: 2.5g
Low GI

**These parcels are so pretty on the plate and they're packed with delicious vegetables and juicy prawns. If you can't find spring greens, you can use dark green cabbage leaves instead. It's worth investing in some top-quality balsamic vinegar: a little goes a long way, as it's really syrupy and highly flavoured – and a teaspoon has only 4 calories.**

4 large spring green (collard green) leaves, trimmed

2 baby courgettes (zucchini), cut into thin matchsticks

2 small carrots, cut into thin matchsticks

50g/1¾oz baby asparagus tips, trimmed

2 spring onions (scallions), sliced

100g/3½oz cooked peeled prawns (shrimp)

2 tbsp chopped fresh parsley

grated zest and juice of ½ lemon

salt and freshly ground black pepper

200g/7oz ripe tomatoes, peeled

few drops of balsamic vinegar, for drizzling (optional)

Serves 2
Prep: 15 minutes
Cook: 10-12 minutes

Dip the spring green leaves into a large saucepan of salted boiling water for about 30 seconds to blanch them. Remove immediately and plunge into cold water, then drain well and pat dry with kitchen paper.

Spread the leaves out on a clean work surface. Divide the courgettes, carrots, asparagus, spring onions and prawns between the leaves. Sprinkle the parsley, lemon zest and juice over the top, then season with a little salt and pepper.

Fold the leaves around the filling and roll up, tucking in the sides securely to seal the 'parcels'.

Arrange the parcels, seam-side underneath, in a colander or the top of a steamer and place over a saucepan of simmering water. Cover with a tight-fitting lid and steam for 10–12 minutes, or until the vegetables are cooked and tender.

Meanwhile, cut the tomatoes in half and scoop out and discard the seeds. Blitz the tomato flesh to a purée in a blender and season lightly with salt and pepper.

Serve the hot parcels in a pool of puréed tomatoes, and drizzle with balsamic vinegar, if you like.

# CHUNKY MINESTRONE

**Eat this substantial soup for a healthy lunch, or serve it with crusty bread (an average 60g/2¼oz serving will be 150 calories and 1g fat) or a salad for your main meal. You can double the quantities given and keep the minestrone in the refrigerator for a few days, or freeze some in individual portions for later use.**

1 onion, chopped

1 leek, chopped

2 garlic cloves, crushed

2 celery sticks, chopped

1 carrot, chopped

750ml/1¼ pints/3 cups vegetable stock

2 large tomatoes, peeled and chopped

1 bay leaf

few fresh thyme sprigs

salt and freshly ground black pepper

100g/3½oz canned cannellini beans, rinsed and drained

100g/3½oz spring greens (collard greens), shredded

15g/½oz dried vermicelli (1 coil)

2 tbsp chopped fresh parsley

Serves 2

Prep: 15 minutes

Cook: 1¼ hours

Put the onion, leek, garlic, celery, carrot and stock in a large saucepan. Place over a high heat, cover the pan and bring to the boil. Boil hard for 5 minutes, then uncover the pan, reduce the heat to low and simmer for 20 minutes, or until the vegetables are tender.

Add the tomatoes, bay leaf and thyme. Season with salt and pepper and simmer for 20 minutes.

Add the cannellini beans and continue simmering gently for about 15 minutes. Stir in the spring greens and vermicelli and cook for 10 minutes, or until the pasta is tender.

Check the seasoning and remove the bay leaf. Divide the hot soup between two serving bowls, sprinkle with parsley and serve immediately.

OR TRY THIS…
MAKE THE MINESTRONE MORE SUBSTANTIAL BY ADDING 125G/4½OZ DICED POTATO WITH THE CANNELLINI BEANS, WHICH INCREASES THE CALORIE COUNT TO 150 CALORIES PER SERVING. IF YOU SPRINKLE 1 TABLESPOON GRATED PARMESAN CHEESE OVER YOUR BOWL OF SOUP, YOU'LL ADD 40 CALORIES AND 3G FAT.

Per serving
100 kcals
Fat: 0.5g
Fibre: 9g
Medium GI

# HOT AND SOUR CHICKEN SOUP

**Even though it's only 100 calories, this really is a meal in a bowl…and a very attractive one, too. If you like aromatic, spicy Thai food, you'll love this soup. And what's even better, it takes only 30 minutes to make from start to finish. You can use regular button or chestnut mushrooms if you don't have shiitake.**

spray oil

8 spring onions (scallions), sliced

1 garlic clove, crushed

1 tbsp finely chopped fresh root ginger

1 red bird's eye (Thai) chilli, diced

200g/7oz skinned chicken breast fillets, thinly sliced

100g/3½oz fresh shiitake mushrooms, sliced

1 litre/1¾ pints/4 cups hot vegetable stock

200g/7oz spring greens (collard greens) or pak choi, shredded

100g/3½oz/1 cup bean sprouts

1 tbsp dark soy sauce

1 tbsp nam pla (Thai fish sauce)

1 tbsp rice vinegar

2 tbsp chopped fresh coriander (cilantro)

Serves 4

Prep: 15 minutes

Cook: 15 minutes

Lightly spray a large saucepan with oil and place over a medium heat. When it's hot, add the spring onions, garlic, ginger, chilli, chicken and mushrooms. Stir-fry for 3–4 minutes until the vegetables are starting to colour and the chicken is sealed all over and golden brown.

Add the hot vegetable stock and bring to the boil. Reduce the heat and simmer gently for 5 minutes.

Add the spring greens and simmer for a further 5 minutes, or until the chicken is cooked right through.

Stir in the bean sprouts, soy sauce, nam pla and vinegar. Ladle the soup into four bowls, sprinkle with chopped coriander and serve piping hot.

Per serving
100 kcals
Fat: 1.5g
Fibre: 2.5g
Low GI

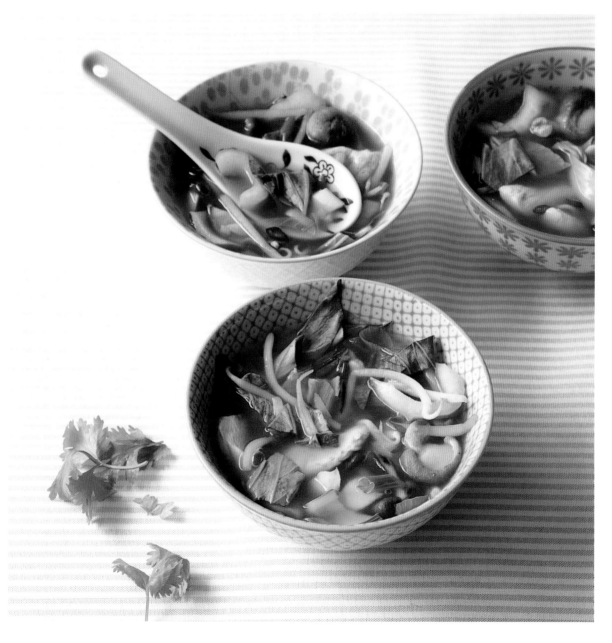

# FRUITY FILO STACKS

Different brands of filo pastry come in varying sizes and you can buy fresh or frozen filo pastry. You can always freeze any unused sheets for another occasion. If you brush the sheets with beaten egg instead of the more usual melted butter, it will have a fraction of the calories but still taste fabulous. We've used fresh raspberries and apricots for this summer dessert, but you could try strawberries or redcurrants and two fresh peaches instead.

4 x 15g/½oz sheets filo pastry (dough)
1 small egg, beaten
225g/8oz/1 cup 0% fat Greek yogurt
4 ripe apricots, stoned and quartered
125g/4½oz/1 cup raspberries
1 tsp icing (confectioners') sugar, sifted, for dusting

Serves 4
Prep: 20 minutes
Cook: 8–10 minutes

Preheat the oven to 200°C/400°F/Gas mark 6.

Place a sheet of filo pastry on a clean work surface. Brush with a little beaten egg and cover with another sheet. Brush and layer in this way until all the sheets are used up. Brush the top sheet with beaten egg.

Cut the filo pastry rectangle into three long strips. Cut each strip into four squares – you should end up with 12 squares. Transfer to a non-stick baking tray and bake for 8–10 minutes, or until crisp and golden. Leave to cool.

Spread a layer of yogurt over one of the filo sheets and place two pieces of apricots and a few raspberries on top. Cover with another sheet, spread with yogurt and add two more apricots and some raspberries. Top the stack with a third filo sheet.

Assemble three more stacks in the same way. Dust lightly with sifted icing sugar and serve immediately.

Per serving
100 kcals
Fat: 3.5g
Fibre: 0.7g
Medium GI

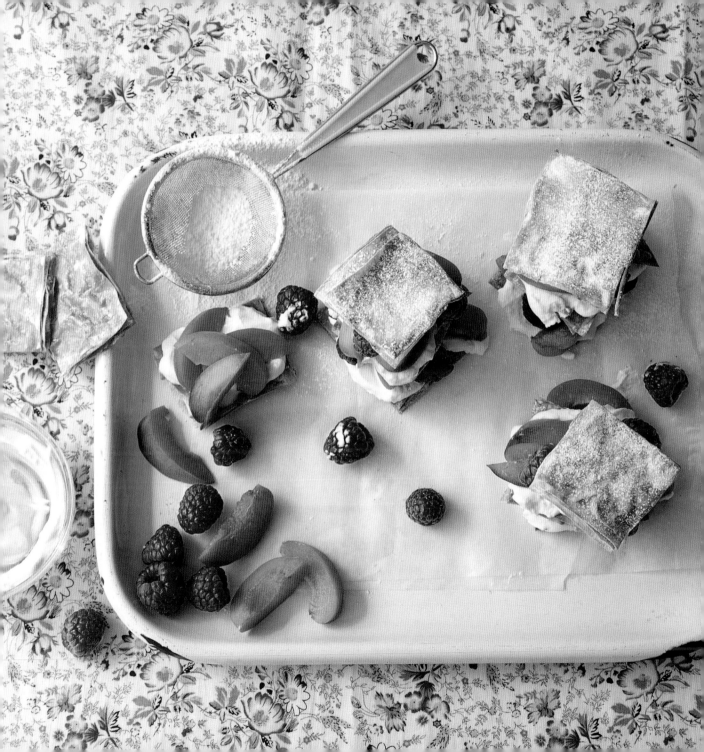

# AMARETTI SUMMER FRUIT MERINGUE

**Small and intensely flavoured, amaretti are made from bitter-tasting almonds. Don't be tempted to use more in this recipe, as a single 4g biscuit (cookie) contains 17 calories. They are available in most good supermarkets as well as Italian delis.**

3 medium plums, stoned and cut into quarters
1 tsp soft brown sugar
pinch of ground ginger
85g/3oz/generous ⅔ cup fresh or frozen raspberries
1 egg white
2 tsp caster (superfine) sugar
3 amaretti biscuits (cookies), roughly crushed

Serves 2
Prep: 15 minutes
Cook: 15–20 minutes

Preheat the oven to 180°C/350°F/Gas mark 4.

Put the plums in a small saucepan with the brown sugar, ginger and a little water. Bring to the boil, stirring occasionally until the sugar dissolves, and then simmer very gently over a low heat for about 10 minutes, or until the plums are tender. Stir in the raspberries and remove from the heat.

Whisk the egg white in a clean, dry bowl until stiff. Add the caster sugar and continue whisking until stiff and glossy.

Divide the amaretti biscuits between two individual ramekin dishes. Cover with the cooked fruit and then spoon the meringue on top.

Bake for about 8 minutes, or until the meringue is set and golden brown. Serve immediately.

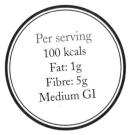

Per serving
100 kcals
Fat: 1g
Fibre: 5g
Medium GI

OR TRY THIS...
INSTEAD OF PLUMS, USE OTHER STONE FRUITS, SUCH AS FRESH GREENGAGES OR APRICOTS. THE CALORIES WILL STAY THE SAME.

# AFFOGATO AL CAFFE

**This has to be the quickest and easiest dessert ever. If you are a coffee addict, you will just love it – the combination of icy cold creamy ice cream and hot bitter espresso is sublime. If you are serving it late in the evening, you could use decaffeinated coffee. Don't be tempted to cheat and use regular vanilla ice cream – the same size scoop could add a whopping 150 calories!**

2 small cups extremely hot, freshly made espresso coffee

2 x 125ml/4fl oz/½ cup scoops low-fat vanilla ice cream

2 x 4g/⅛oz amaretti biscuits (cookies), to serve

Serves 2
Prep: 5 minutes
Cook: 5 minutes

Make the coffee using an espresso maker if you have one. It's essential that it's really strong and piping hot.

Scoop a neat ball of ice-cold low-fat vanilla ice cream into each bowl or cup. The ice cream should be frozen really hard so that it does not melt as soon as the espresso is added.

Pour the hot espresso over the ice cream and eat immediately, before the ice cream melts into the coffee. Serve with the amaretti biscuits.

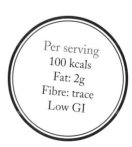

Per serving
100 kcals
Fat: 2g
Fibre: trace
Low GI

# FROZEN BERRIES WITH WHITE CHOCOLATE

**The white chocolate looks amazing drizzled over the colourful frozen berries. Whether you use dark, milk or white chocolate, the calories are practically the same, although white and milk chocolate have one more gram of fat per 25g/¾oz than dark (9g as opposed to 8g).**

400g/14oz/2¾ cups mixed berries, such as raspberries, blueberries, blackberries, strawberries

60g/2¼oz white chocolate, broken into pieces

4 tbsp virtually fat-free fromage frais

Serves 4
Prep: 5 minutes
Freeze: 20 minutes
Cook: 1 minute

Spread out the berries on a plate or baking sheet or divide them between four glasses. Put them in the freezer for 20 minutes until they are slightly frozen but not solid.

Just before serving, put the white chocolate pieces into a microwave-proof basin or jug. Microwave on High for 1 minute and then stir in the fromage frais. Alternatively, you can melt the chocolate in a heatproof basin set over a saucepan of simmering water.

Serve the frozen berries drizzled with the hot white chocolate sauce.

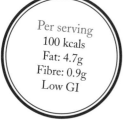

Per serving
100 kcals
Fat: 4.7g
Fibre: 0.9g
Low GI

OR TRY THIS...
DIVIDE 400G/14OZ/2¾ CUPS FRESH HULLED STRAWBERRIES AMONG FOUR PLATES. POUR THE HOT WHITE CHOCOLATE SAUCE INTO FOUR SMALL RAMEKINS AND USE AS A DIP FOR THE BERRIES.

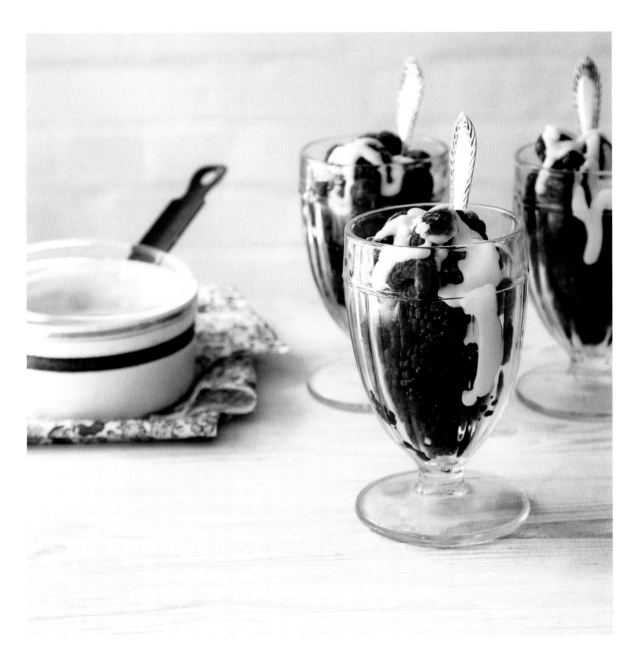

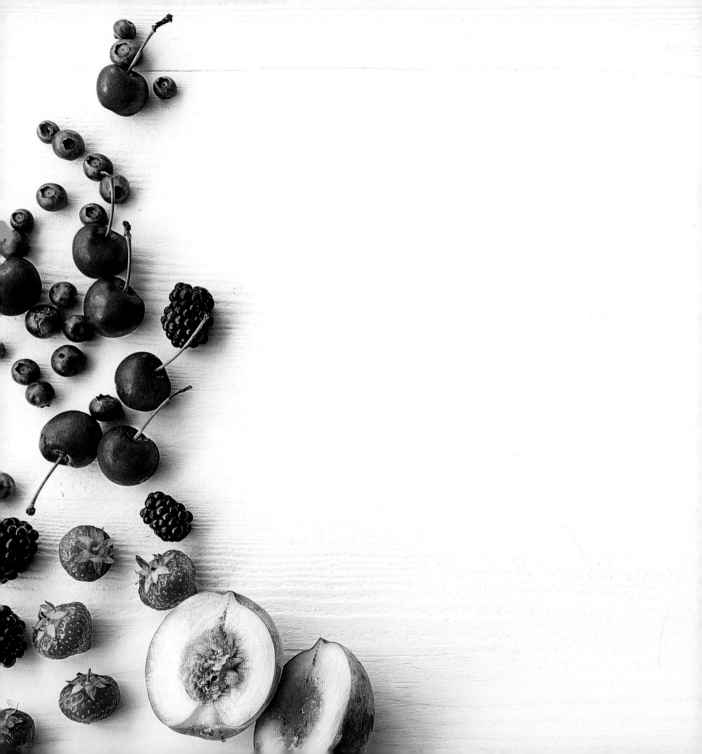

# 200 calories

# CINNAMON FRENCH TOAST WITH BERRIES

**French toast tastes just as good, if not better, with fruit and fromage frais as it does with maple syrup, which has 52 calories per tablespoon – and most of us add far more than that! This is not only delicious for breakfast or brunch, it can be eaten as a dessert, too.**

1 large free-range egg
4 tbsp skimmed (lowfat) milk
good pinch of ground cinnamon
pinch of soft brown sugar
2 medium-cut slices multi-grain bread
spray oil

**To serve**
4 tbsp virtually fat-free fromage frais
150g/5½oz/1 cup sliced ripe strawberries and blueberries

Serves 2
Prep: 5 minutes
Soak: 5 minutes
Cook: 4–6 minutes

Beat the egg, milk, cinnamon and sugar together in a shallow bowl.

Place the slices of bread in the bowl and leave for about 5 minutes, or until the bread has soaked up all the egg mixture.

Lightly spray a non-stick frying pan with oil and place over a low heat. Add the soaked bread and cook gently for 2–3 minutes on each side until golden brown all over.

Place the French toast on two warmed serving plates and serve immediately with the fromage frais and fresh berries.

Per serving
200 kcals
Fat: 6g
Fibre: 1.8g
Medium GI

OR TRY THIS...
USE FRESH RASPBERRIES INSTEAD OF STRAWBERRIES OR BLUEBERRIES, AND SUBSTITUTE 0% FAT NATURAL GREEK YOGURT FOR THE FROMAGE FRAIS AT NO EXTRA CALORIES.

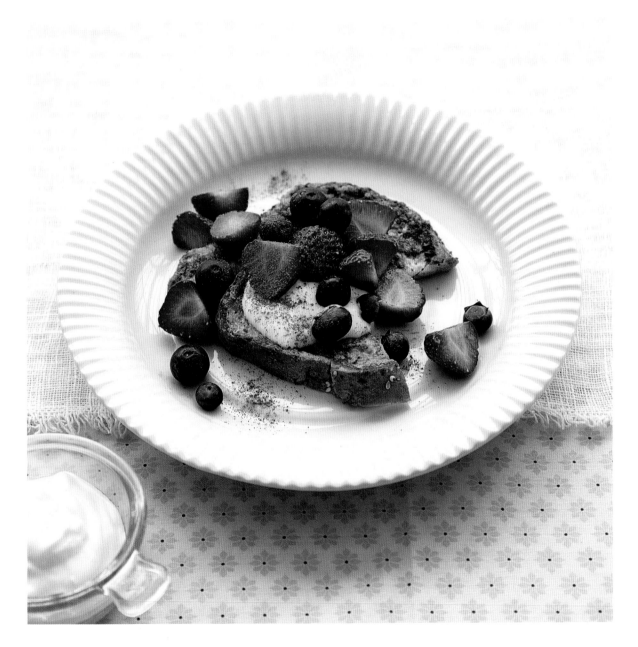

# BREAKFAST
# BLT TOASTIE

**The average BLT is high in fat and calories, but you can enjoy this classic sandwich for only 200 calories by using very lean bacon and extra-light mayonnaise. A heaped teaspoon of mayonnaise can vary from as much as 80 calories and 9g fat to as little as 32 calories and 3g for reduced-calorie, or 12 calories (no fat) for extra-light. It pays to be a canny shopper when you're watching your waistline.**

4 lean extra-thin rashers (slices) back
(Canadian) bacon, all visible fat removed
1 tomato, sliced
4 medium-cut slices whole-grain bread
2 tsp tomato ketchup
2 tsp extra-light mayonnaise
few crisp lettuce leaves
freshly ground black pepper

Serves 2
Prep: 5 minutes
Cook: 5 minutes

Preheat the grill (broiler). Cook the bacon and tomato slices under the hot grill or in a frying pan that has been sprayed lightly with oil for 4–5 minutes until the bacon is crisp and golden brown and the tomato is tender.

Toast the slices of bread on both sides until lightly golden.

Thinly spread two slices of toast with the ketchup and the others with mayonnaise.

Arrange the lettuce leaves on top of the mayonnaise-covered toast and top with the grilled tomato and bacon. Season with freshly ground black pepper and cover with the ketchup-spread toast. Cut each sandwich in half and eat immediately while the bacon and tomato are still warm.

Per serving
200 kcals
Fat: 5g
Fibre: 3g
Medium GI

# GRANOLA BERRY BREAKFAST BOWL

**If you have a sweet tooth you can use fat-free strawberry or raspberry yogurt instead of plain yogurt – the calories and fat grams will stay the same. Always check the labels carefully when buying packets of granola because some brands are much higher in fat and sugar than others.**

50g/1¾oz/scant ½ cup low-fat granola
200g/7oz/scant 1 cup very low-fat plain yogurt
300g/10½oz/2 cups mixed fresh berries, such as strawberries, blueberries, raspberries, redcurrants

Serves 2
Prep: 10 minutes

Put half of the granola into two glass bowls, then cover the granola with half of the yogurt and half the berries.

Add the remaining granola and then the rest of the yogurt. Top with a layer of berries and eat immediately.

Per serving
200 kcals
Fat: 1.5g
Fibre: 5g
Medium GI

OR TRY THIS...
INSTEAD OF FRESH BERRIES, YOU CAN TOP EACH BOWL OF GRANOLA AND YOGURT WITH ONE SLICED OR CUBED FRESH PEACH OR NECTARINE, OR HALF A SMALL BANANA, THINLY SLICED. THE CALORIES PER SERVING WILL REMAIN THE SAME.

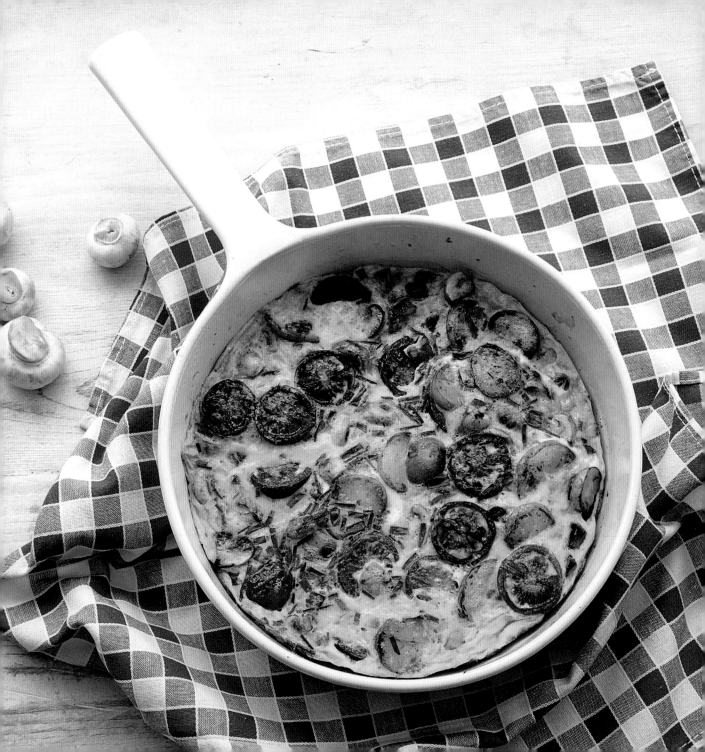

# ALL-DAY BREAKFAST OMELETTE

Per serving
200 kcals
Fat: 13.5g
Fibre: 1.2g
Medium GI

**This is a really easy breakfast – everything is cooked together in the same pan. In fact, it's so delicious and low in calories that you'll probably enjoy eating it at any time of day. It's also a great way of using up leftover cooked potatoes.**

spray olive oil
60g/2¼oz cooked new potatoes, diced
100g/3½oz button (white) mushrooms, quartered
30g/1oz lean thin-cut rashers (slices) back (Canadian) bacon, all visible fat removed, chopped
8 cherry tomatoes, halved
3 medium free-range eggs
2 tbsp water
salt and freshly ground black pepper
1 tbsp snipped fresh chives

Serves 2
Prep: 5 minutes
Cook: 15 minutes

Lightly spray a large, non-stick, ovenproof frying pan with oil and place over a medium heat. When it's hot, add the potatoes, mushrooms and bacon and cook for 5 minutes, turning occasionally, until the vegetables are golden brown and the bacon is crisping up. Add the cherry tomatoes and continue cooking for 2–3 minutes.

Beat the eggs and water together in a bowl. Season lightly with salt and pepper and beat in the chives.

Preheat the grill (broiler). Pour the beaten egg into the frying pan around the bacon and vegetables. Reduce the heat to low and cook gently for 4–5 minutes until the omelette is set and golden brown underneath.

To set and brown the top of the omelette, pop the frying pan under the hot grill for 2–3 minutes. Cut the omelette in half and slide out onto two serving plates. Eat immediately.

# INDIAN SPICED DHAL SOUP

**Lentils are a great source of protein and fibre and just a few go a long way in this delicious and filling soup; it really is a meal in a bowl. You can make double the quantity and freeze individual portions for a later date. Use the small red or orange lentils rather than green or Puy ones – they won't break up and thicken the soup.**

spray oil
1 small onion, finely chopped
2 celery sticks, diced
1 leek, chopped
100g/3½oz carrot, diced
1 tsp finely chopped fresh root ginger
2 garlic cloves, crushed
1 tsp black mustard seeds
1 tsp hot chilli powder
1 tsp ground cumin
1 tsp turmeric
85g/3oz/scant ½ cup split red lentils
600ml/1 pint/2½ cups vegetable stock
salt and freshly ground black pepper
1 small bunch of fresh coriander
(cilantro), chopped

Spray a large saucepan lightly with oil and set over a low heat. Add the onion, celery, leek, carrot, ginger and garlic and cook, stirring occasionally, for about 10 minutes until starting to soften.

Stir in the mustard seeds and cook for 2 minutes, or until they start to pop. Add the chilli, cumin, turmeric and lentils and cook for 1 minute.

Add the vegetable stock, turn up the heat and bring to the boil. Reduce the heat and simmer gently for about 15 minutes, or until the vegetables are tender and the lentils have broken down to thicken the soup.

Season to taste with a little salt and freshly ground black pepper and stir in the chopped coriander. Serve immediately.

Serves 2
Prep: 10 minutes
Cook: 30 minutes

OR TRY THIS...
IF YOU PREFER A SMOOTHER RESULT, YOU CAN BLITZ THIS SOUP IN A BLENDER OR FOOD PROCESSOR.

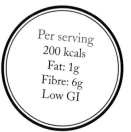

Per serving
200 kcals
Fat: 1g
Fibre: 6g
Low GI

# SPICED WINTER ROOTS SOUP

**The carrots, parsnips and swede thicken this soup naturally, giving it a lovely texture and vibrant colour. Root vegetables are quite high in starch and sugar and should always be eaten in moderation.**

spray oil
1 onion, finely chopped
2 celery sticks, chopped
200g/7oz carrots, thinly sliced
175g/6oz parsnips, thinly sliced
200g/7oz swede (rutabaga), peeled and cubed
1 garlic clove, crushed
1 tsp ground cumin
1 tsp turmeric
pinch of ground nutmeg
600ml/1 pint/2½ cups vegetable stock
1 bay leaf
grated zest and juice of ½ orange
salt and freshly ground black pepper
2 tbsp chopped fresh parsley
30g/1oz reduced-fat Cheddar cheese, grated, to serve

Serves 2
Prep: 15 minutes
Cook: 30 minutes

Lightly spray a large saucepan with oil and place over a low heat. Add the onion, celery, carrots, parsnips, swede and garlic and cook gently for 10 minutes, or until the vegetables are softened.

Stir in the spices and cook for 1 minute. Add the vegetable stock and bay leaf and bring to the boil. Reduce the heat and simmer gently for 15 minutes, or until all the vegetables are cooked and tender. Remove the bay leaf.

Blitz the soup in batches in a blender or food processor until smooth. Return to the same pan and stir in the orange zest and juice. Season to taste with salt and pepper, add the parsley and reheat gently until the soup is piping hot.

Ladle the soup into serving bowls and serve hot, sprinkled with the grated cheese.

Per serving
200 kcals
Fat: 3.5g
Fibre: 10g
Medium GI

# PUMPKIN SOUP WITH TORTILLA CHIPS

A warming substantial soup that tastes and looks amazing. It's great in the autumn when pumpkins are plentiful and in season – serve it at Hallowe'en or for a bonfire night party. Measure out the tortilla chips carefully and check the nutritional information on the packet before buying, as the calorie and fat content can vary significantly depending on the brand.

spray oil
1 onion, thinly sliced
2 garlic cloves, crushed
1 tsp smoked paprika
675g/1½lb pumpkin, peeled, deseeded and cubed
750ml/1¼ pints/3 cups hot vegetable stock
60ml/2fl oz/¼ cup low-fat crème fraîche
freshly ground black pepper

**To serve**
few fresh chives, snipped
45g/1½oz plain tortilla chips, roughly crushed
60g/2¼oz/¼ cup coarsely grated low-fat Cheddar cheese

Serves 4
Prep: 15 minutes
Cook: 30–35 minutes

Spray a large pan lightly with oil and place over a very low heat. Add the onion and garlic and cook very gently, stirring occasionally to prevent them sticking to the pan, for about 15 minutes, or until tender and starting to caramelize. Stir in the paprika.

Add the pumpkin and hot stock and bring to the boil. Reduce the heat to a simmer, cover the pan and cook gently for 15–20 minutes, or until the pumpkin is tender.

Blitz the soup in a blender or purée in the pan with a hand-held electric blender until really smooth. Stir in the crème fraîche and season to taste with pepper.

Ladle the hot soup into bowls and serve immediately, sprinkled with chives, tortilla chips and grated cheese.

Per serving
200 kcals
Fat: 7.5g
Fibre: 3.5g
Medium GI

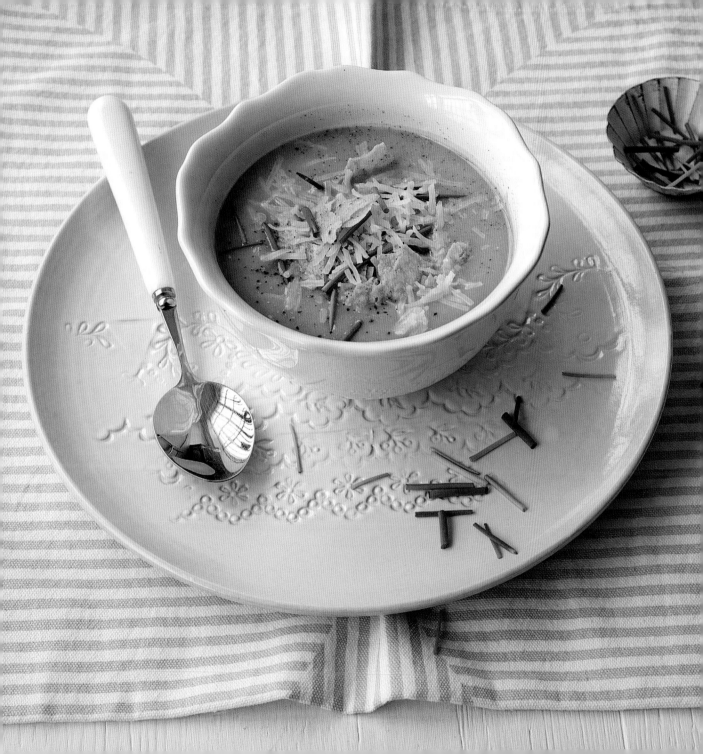

# PRAWN AND ROCKET LINGUINE

**Raw prawns (shrimp) are now available at most fresh fish counters in supermarkets or in packets in the frozen food aisles. Always defrost them thoroughly before cooking. Take care not to overcook them, or they will become tough and dry. They cook perfectly to a juicy succulence in about 3–4 minutes – as soon as they turn pink they are ready to eat. You can use cooked prawns, but the flavour won't be as good.**

100g/3½oz dried linguine
spray oil
2 garlic cloves, crushed
pinch of dried hot chilli flakes
juice of 1 lime
85ml/3fl oz/scant ⅓ cup dry white wine
200g/7oz peeled raw tiger prawns (jumbo shrimp)
a large handful of wild rocket (arugula)
salt and freshly ground black pepper

Serves 2
Prep: 5 minutes
Cook: 8–12 minutes

Cook the linguine in a large saucepan of salted boiling water according to the packet instructions until just tender (al dente). Drain well.

While the pasta is cooking, lightly spray a large frying pan with oil and place over a low heat. Add the garlic and cook, without browning, for 1 minute.

Add the chilli flakes and stir well. Pour in the lime juice and wine, then turn up the heat and let it bubble away for about 5 minutes until reduced and concentrated.

Add the prawns and cook for 1–2 minutes until pink underneath, then turn them over and cook the other side. Do not overcook them, or they will be less juicy and succulent.

Gently toss the prawn mixture and rocket with the cooked linguine. Add a little salt and a good grinding of pepper. Divide between two warmed deep serving plates and serve immediately.

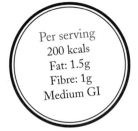

Per serving
200 kcals
Fat: 1.5g
Fibre: 1g
Medium GI

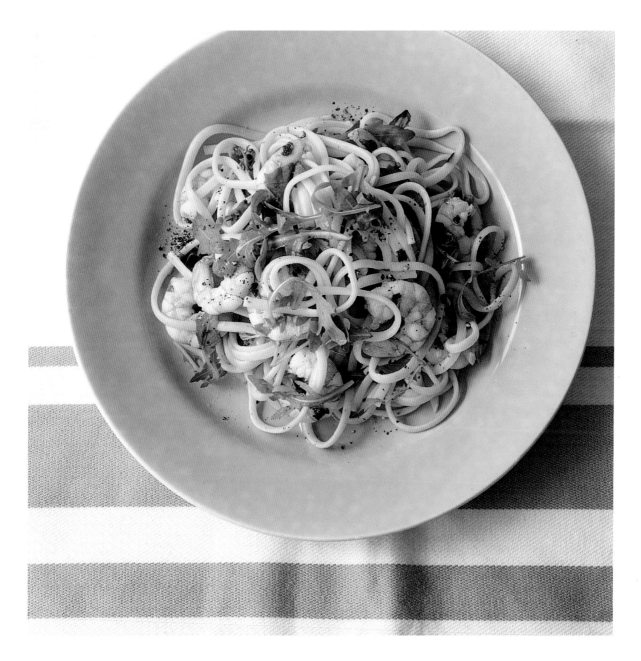

# TOMATO AND ROCKET FRITTATA

**This frittata is surprisingly filling and you can eat it for breakfast, lunch or dinner. Alternatively, make it the evening before and wrap in clingfilm (plastic wrap) to take a portion to work for a delicious packed lunch, or to enjoy as part of a picnic. It's great cold and easy to eat with your fingers.**

spray olive oil
1 red onion, thinly sliced
2 garlic cloves, crushed
2 courgettes (zucchini), thinly sliced
2 ripe tomatoes, chopped
4 medium free-range eggs
salt and freshly ground black pepper
handful of wild rocket (arugula), torn,
plus extra to serve
few fresh basil or parsley sprigs, chopped

Serves 2
Prep: 10 minutes
Cook: 25–30 minutes

Lightly spray a large, non-stick, ovenproof frying pan with oil and set over a very low heat. Add the onion and garlic and cook gently for 10–15 minutes, stirring occasionally to prevent them sticking to the pan, until the onion starts to caramelize. Add the courgettes and tomatoes and cook for a further 5 minutes.

Preheat the grill (broiler). Beat the eggs in a bowl and season with a little salt and pepper. Stir in the rocket and chopped herbs.

Pour the egg mixture over the vegetables in the frying pan and cook gently for 15 minutes until the frittata is set and golden underneath but still slightly runny on top.

Pop the pan under the hot grill for 2–3 minutes until the top is set and golden brown.

Slide the frittata out of the pan onto a plate and cut in half. Serve hot, lukewarm or cold with some fresh rocket.

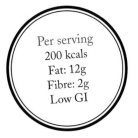

Per serving
200 kcals
Fat: 12g
Fibre: 2g
Low GI

OR TRY THIS...
USE BABY SPINACH LEAVES INSTEAD OF
THE ROCKET; THEIR FLAVOUR IS MILDER
AND LESS PEPPERY.

# WARM CRUNCHY ASPARAGUS AND PRAWN SALAD

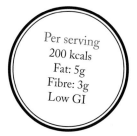

Per serving
200 kcals
Fat: 5g
Fibre: 3g
Low GI

**The dressing on these crunchy vegetables and prawns can be used for other Thai and Asian salads. Reduced-fat coconut milk is sold in cans in most supermarkets as well as in Asian stores. Don't use full-fat coconut milk or creamed coconut instead – it has almost double the calories and fat grams.**

150g/5½oz asparagus, cut in half

115g/4oz mangetout (snow peas)

250g/9oz cooked peeled king prawns (shrimp)

100g/3½oz mixed rocket (arugula), watercress and spinach

1 red bird's eye (Thai) chilli, finely diced

few fresh coriander (cilantro) sprigs, roughly chopped

**Spicy coconut dressing**

50ml/1¾fl oz/scant ¼ cup reduced-fat coconut milk

2 tsp nam pla (Thai fish sauce)

juice of 1 lime

Serves 2

Prep: 10 minutes

Cook: 5 minutes

Cook the asparagus in a saucepan of boiling salted water for 3–4 minutes until it is just tender but retains a little 'bite' and is still a lovely bright green colour. Drain well.

Cook the mangetout in another saucepan of boiling water for 2 minutes – it should be bright green and still crisp. Drain well.

Make the spicy coconut dressing: gently heat the coconut milk in a small saucepan. Stir in the nam pla and lime juice and remove from the heat.

Mix the asparagus, mangetout, prawns, mixed leaves, chilli and coriander together in a salad bowl. Pour over the warm dressing and gently toss everything together. Serve immediately.

OR TRY THIS...
SUGAR SNAP PEAS MAKE A CRUNCHY ALTERNATIVE TO MANGETOUT. JUST TRIM AND STRING THEM IF NECESSARY, AND THEN COOK IN BOILING WATER FOR 2 MINUTES.

# MEXICAN CHICKEN TORTILLA BASKETS

**The tortilla baskets look so attractive and add some crunch to this Mexican chicken salad. If you're just making enough for two, it's better to buy low-fat guacamole than make it yourself. Avocados are a healthy but high-fat food, and even baby ones pack a whopping 200 calories and 18g fat.**

spray oil
2 x 30g/1oz soft tortillas
4 ripe cherry tomatoes, halved
½ yellow (bell) pepper, deseeded and chopped
2 spring onions (scallions), chopped
30g/1oz baby salad leaves
125g/4½oz cooked skinned chicken breast, diced
2 tbsp low-fat guacamole
2 tbsp chopped fresh coriander (cilantro)

**For the spicy orange dressing**
1 tbsp oil-free vinaigrette dressing
grated zest and juice of ½ orange
½ red chilli, deseeded and finely diced

Serves 2
Prep: 15 minutes
Cook: 8–10 minutes

Preheat the oven to 200°C/400°F/Gas mark 6.

Lightly spray two Yorkshire-pudding moulds or tartlet tins with oil. Press the tortillas down into the moulds to make a basket shape and cook in the oven for 8–10 minutes until crisp and golden. Check that they do not over-brown. Remove from the oven and leave to cool.

Blend the dressing ingredients together in a small bowl or shake them in a screwtop jar until well combined.

Mix the tomatoes, yellow pepper, spring onions, salad leaves and chicken together in another bowl, then add the dressing and toss gently until everything is lightly dressed.

Divide the chicken salad mixture between the tortilla baskets and top each one with a spoonful of guacamole and some chopped coriander.

Per serving
200 kcals
Fat: 2.9g
Fibre: 2.1g
Medium GI

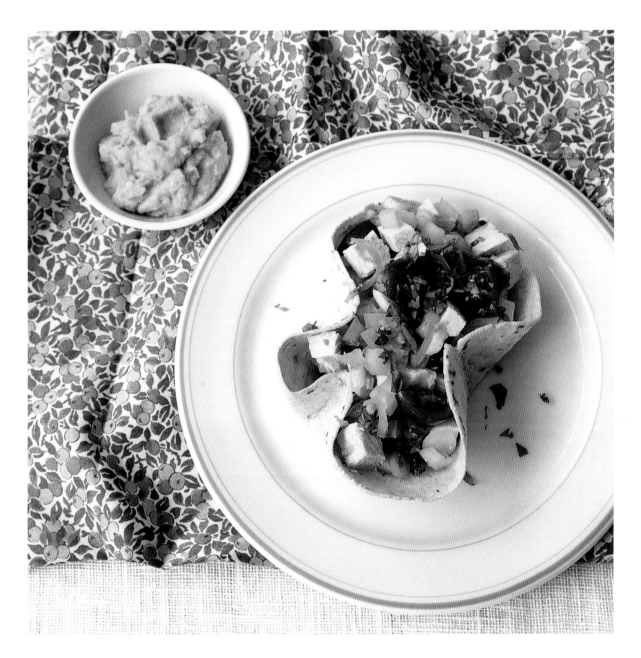

# WARM SCALLOP, BACON AND ROCKET SALAD

**Scallops are very 'meaty' and low in fat, but take care not to overcook them, or they will lose their juicy tenderness. If your scallops come with coral attached, leave it on and allow to cook for a little longer.**

4 lean extra-thin rashers (slices) back (Canadian) bacon, all visible fat removed
8 large scallops
70g/2½oz wild rocket (arugula)
4 spring onions (scallions), chopped
6 baby plum tomatoes, halved
few fresh parsley sprigs, finely chopped
2 tbsp oil-free vinaigrette dressing
grated zest and juice of 1 lemon
salt and freshly ground black pepper
fresh chives, snipped, to garnish

Serves 2
Prep: 15 minutes
Cook: 5 minutes

Preheat the grill (broiler). Using the blade of a knife, stretch out each bacon rasher lengthways and then cut it in half. Wrap each scallop in a piece of bacon.

Put the scallops on a foil-lined grill pan and cook under the hot grill for about 5 minutes, turning them occasionally, until the scallops are cooked but still tender and the bacon is crisp and golden brown.

While the scallops are cooking, mix the rocket, spring onions, tomatoes and most of the parsley together in a bowl.

Blend the vinaigrette dressing with the lemon zest and juice in a bowl or shake in a screwtop jar until well combined, then add to the salad and toss gently until everything is lightly dressed.

Arrange a pyramid of salad on each serving plate and place the bacon-wrapped scallops on top. Season to taste with a little salt and pepper, then sprinkle with the remaining parsley and snipped chives.

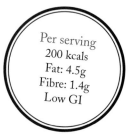

Per serving
200 kcals
Fat: 4.5g
Fibre: 1.4g
Low GI

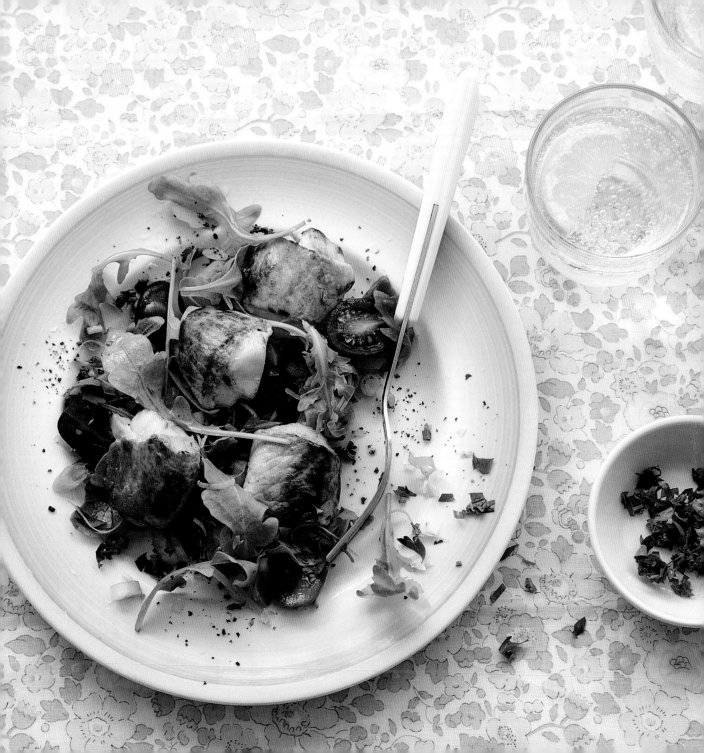

# GRIDDLED HOT SQUID SALAD

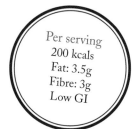

Per serving
200 kcals
Fat: 3.5g
Fibre: 3g
Low GI

**If you are pushed for time, you can ask the fishmonger to clean and prepare the squid for you – many supermarket fresh fish counters sell it ready prepared. Be careful not to overcook it, or it will become tough and chewy and lose its juicy succulence. Cooking squid on a really hot ridged grill pan will add attractive golden brown lines to the white flesh.**

350g/12oz cleaned squid
sea salt and freshly ground black pepper
spray olive oil
handful of fresh mint leaves
handful of fresh basil leaves
2 spring onions (scallions), sliced
¼ red onion, diced
¼ cucumber, halved and sliced
150g/5½oz cherry tomatoes, halved

**For the chilli dressing**
juice of 1 lime
1 tbsp nam pla (Thai fish sauce)
1 small red chilli, deseeded and diced
1 garlic clove, crushed
handful of fresh coriander (cilantro), finely chopped

Serves 2
Prep: 20 minutes
Cook: 2 minutes

Cut each squid sac down one side and open it out flat. Score one side of the flesh in a criss-cross pattern without cutting all the way through. Season lightly with sea salt and freshly ground black pepper.

Lightly spray a ridged griddle pan with oil and place over a high heat. When the pan is very hot, add the squid and cook for just a few seconds on each side, until it is just tender and the pieces start to curl. Remove from the pan immediately and keep warm.

Blend all the dressing ingredients together in a small bowl or shake in a screw-top jar.

Mix the mint and basil leaves with the spring onions, red onion, cucumber and cherry tomatoes in a bowl. Add the squid and the dressing and gently toss everything together. Divide between two serving plates and serve while the squid is still hot.

SLIM FACT...
SQUID IS INEXPENSIVE AND A HEALTHY FOOD FOR SLIMMERS – IT'S HIGH IN PROTEIN AND LOW IN FAT. HOWEVER, TRADITIONAL DEEP-FRIED CALAMARI IN BATTER HAS MORE THAN DOUBLE THE CALORIES AND SIX TIMES AS MUCH FAT, SO GIVE IT A MISS!

# HOT AND SOUR BEEF SALAD

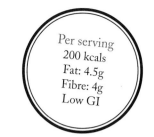

Per serving
200 kcals
Fat: 4.5g
Fibre: 4g
Low GI

**This salad is very refreshing and low in calories if you use really lean steak and remove all the visible fat. You can serve the beef well cooked, medium or rare, depending on how you like it – anything goes as long as it's served hot. The simple dressing can be used on Thai and Vietnamese-style salads.**

200g/7oz lean sirloin steak, all visible fat removed
spray oil
8 spring onions (scallions), trimmed and halved
salt and freshly ground black pepper
¼ cucumber, cut into matchsticks
1 red chilli, deseeded and shredded
50g/1¾oz/½ cup bean sprouts
100g/3½oz baby spinach leaves
few fresh coriander (cilantro), mint and basil sprigs, roughly chopped

**For the Asian dressing**
2 tbsp nam pla (Thai fish sauce)
juice of 1 lime
1 tsp sweet chilli sauce

Serves 2
Prep: 15 minutes
Cook: 5 minutes

In a small bowl, whisk all the dressing ingredients together until well blended.

Cut the steak into thin strips, removing any fat. Lightly spray a ridged griddle pan with oil and place over a high heat.

When the pan is hot, add the steak strips and the spring onions and cook for 2–4 minutes, turning them frequently. The steak should be seared and browned outside but pink and juicy inside, depending on how well cooked you like it. Season with salt and pepper.

Toss the cucumber, chilli, bean sprouts, spinach leaves and chopped herbs in the prepared dressing.

Add the griddled spring onions and steak and toss again until everything is lightly dressed. Eat the salad immediately while it's hot.

OR TRY THIS...
YOU CAN USE REALLY LEAN RUMP STEAK INSTEAD OF SIRLOIN AS LONG AS YOU CAREFULLY REMOVE ALL THE FAT BEFORE CUTTING IT INTO STRIPS.

# CHICORY, PEAR AND ROQUEFORT SALAD

**This is a delicious salad in winter when you fancy something more substantial than lettuce. It's very good at Christmas served with some cold leftover skinned turkey breast (30 calories per 30g/1oz).**

2 heads white or red chicory (Belgian endive), sliced thinly into rounds
1 medium ripe pear, cored and thinly sliced
¼ red onion, finely chopped
1 ripe baby avocado, peeled, stoned and diced
30g/1oz Roquefort cheese, diced
small bunch of parsley, finely chopped
3 tbsp oil-free vinaigrette dressing
1 tsp honey mustard
juice of 1 lemon
salt and freshly ground black pepper

Serves 2
Prep: 10 minutes

Mix the chicory, pear, onion, avocado, Roquefort and parsley together in a bowl.

Blend the dressing with the mustard and lemon juice and season with salt and pepper; either whisk together in a bowl or shake together in a screwtop jar until emulsified.

Pour the dressing over the salad and toss gently together. Serve immediately.

Per serving
200 kcals
Fat: 14g
Fibre: 3g
Low GI

OR TRY THIS...
INSTEAD OF A PEAR, USE A MEDIUM-SIZED JUICY RED-SKINNED APPLE, SUCH AS COX'S OR BRAEBURN. CORE AND CUT INTO SMALL CHUNKS. SUBSTITUTE DOLCELATTE FOR ROQUEFORT AND THE CALORIES REMAIN THE SAME. HOWEVER, IF YOU USE STILTON, YOU WILL ADD APPROXIMATELY 10 CALORIES AND 1G FAT PER SERVING.

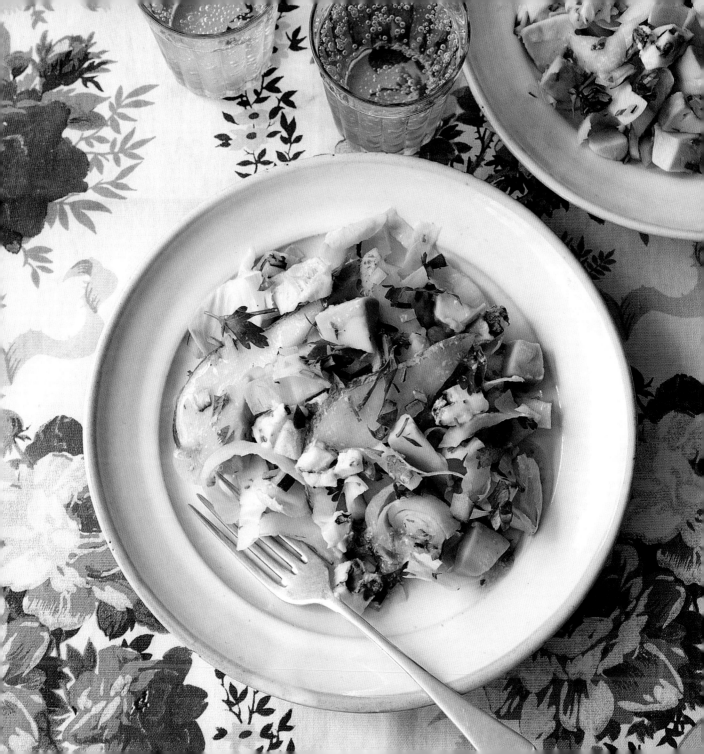

# BARBECUED QUORN AND ASPARAGUS SALAD

**Quorn is a useful and nutritious food for vegetarians who are watching their weight. It's low in fat and there are only 90 calories in 100g/3½oz plain Quorn. It's also very versatile and can be grilled, threaded onto kebabs or added to stir-fries. You can also buy Quorn mince to make a vegetarian version of spaghetti Bolognese.**

spray olive oil
250g/9oz plain Quorn fillets or pieces
150g/5½oz asparagus, trimmed
200g/7oz courgettes (zucchini), sliced lengthways
1 green (bell) pepper, deseeded and cut into chunks
6 spring onions (scallions), trimmed
50g/1¾oz wild rocket (arugula) leaves
50g/1¾oz baby spinach leaves
2 tbsp oil-free vinaigrette dressing
juice of ½ lime
few drops of balsamic vinegar or soy sauce
few fresh coriander (cilantro) sprigs, roughly chopped
freshly ground black pepper

Serves 2
Prep: 15 minutes
Cook: 10 minutes

Preheat a barbecue or large non-stick griddle pan. It's important that it gets very hot before you start cooking. Spray lightly with oil.

Place the Quorn fillets on the hot grill and cook for 8–10 minutes, turning them frequently, without burning – but don't worry if they are slightly charred.

While the Quorn is cooking, add the asparagus, courgettes, green pepper and spring onions to the hot grill and cook for 6–7 minutes, turning them occasionally, until just tender. Remove and keep warm.

Mix the rocket and spinach together and divide between two serving plates.

Toss the grilled Quorn and vegetables in the dressing and place on top of the salad leaves. Sprinkle with lime juice and drizzle a little balsamic vinegar over the top. Sprinkle with chopped coriander and grind over some pepper. Serve immediately while the salad is warm.

OR TRY THIS...
USE 200G/7OZ RAW JUMBO PRAWNS (SHRIMP) OR CHICKEN BREAST FILLET STRIPS INSTEAD OF QUORN. PRAWNS WILL COOK IN 3–4 MINUTES; CHICKEN WILL TAKE APPROXIMATELY THE SAME TIME AS THE QUORN. THE CALORIES AND FAT GRAMS STAY THE SAME, BUT THE FIBRE WILL BE 5G LESS PER PORTION.

Per serving
200 kcals
Fat: 3.5g
Fibre: 12g
Low GI

# TANDOORI CHICKEN WRAPS

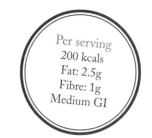

Per serving
200 kcals
Fat: 2.5g
Fibre: 1g
Medium GI

**As when buying tortillas or wraps, check the labels carefully on packets of ready-made chapatis. You are looking for ones with 95 calories and 1.5g fat, or thereabouts. Some brands are much higher, especially flavoured ones made with fat. The tomato salad accompaniment is a traditional Indian kachumber.**

1 tbsp tandoori paste

85g/3oz/scant ⅓ cup low-fat plain yogurt

100g/3½oz chicken breast fillets, cubed

2 x 40g/1½oz chapatis

6 baby plum tomatoes, halved

1 fresh red or green chilli, deseeded and diced

few fresh coriander (cilantro) sprigs, chopped

juice of ½ lime

salt and freshly ground black pepper

**For the mint raita**

50g/1¾oz/scant ¼ cup low-fat plain yogurt

few fresh mint sprigs, chopped

⅛ cucumber, peeled and diced

1 tbsp lemon juice

Serves 2

Prep: 15 minutes

Chill: 30 minutes

Cook: 10 minutes

Blend the tandoori paste with the yogurt in a bowl. Stir in the chicken cubes to coat them with the marinade. Cover and leave to chill in the refrigerator for at least 30 minutes.

Make the raita: mix all the ingredients together in a bowl, season to taste with freshly ground black pepper, then cover and chill in the refrigerator.

Preheat the grill (broiler). Put the marinated chicken cubes on a foil-lined grill pan, spooning over any leftover marinade, and cook under the hot grill, turning them frequently, for about 10 minutes, or until the chicken is cooked right through and golden brown.

Warm the chapatis according to the packet instructions. In a bowl, mix the tomatoes, chilli, coriander and lime juice together. Season with salt and pepper, then stir in the hot chicken.

Divide the chicken mixture between the two chapatis. Top with the mint raita, then fold over or roll up and serve.

OR TRY THIS...
USE SKINNED TURKEY BREAST FILLET INSTEAD OF
CHICKEN WITHOUT AFFECTING THE CALORIE COUNT.

# REFRIED BEAN TORTILLA WRAPS

Wraps are very versatile and make great finger food. If eating them as a packed lunch, make them up in advance and just use the tortillas straight from the packet – there's no need to warm them. Always check the labels carefully when you buy tortillas and wraps because they vary enormously in size, weight and calories. In general, the cornmeal and wholewheat varieties have fewer calories than the soft white ones.

1 x 200g/7oz can refried beans
3 spring onions (scallions), chopped
¼ cucumber, diced
few fresh coriander (cilantro) sprigs, chopped
2 x 30g/1oz wholewheat tortillas
handful of shredded iceberg lettuce
2 tbsp low-fat tomato salsa (see page 22)
2 tbsp virtually fat-free fromage frais
lime wedges, to serve

Serves 2
Prep: 10 minutes
Cook: 5 minutes

Preheat the oven to 190°C/375°F/Gas mark 5, if using.

Mix the refried beans with the spring onions, cucumber and coriander in a bowl.

Warm the tortillas on a ridged griddle pan set over a low heat or wrap them loosely in foil and warm them in the oven for 5 minutes.

Pile the shredded lettuce in the centre of each tortilla and top each with the refried bean mixture and a tablespoon each of tomato salsa and fromage frais. Roll up like a cigar or fold the ends in to enclose the filling and then roll up. Serve immediately, with lime wedges.

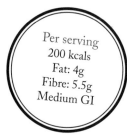

Per serving
200 kcals
Fat: 4g
Fibre: 5.5g
Medium GI

OR TRY THIS...
INSTEAD OF REFRIED BEANS, SUBSTITUTE 150G/5½OZ DICED COOKED CHICKEN BREAST (SKIN REMOVED) OR 125G/4½OZ CANNED TUNA CHUNKS IN BRINE OR SPRING WATER (NOT OIL).
FOR A MORE PEPPERY FLAVOUR, USE WATERCRESS OR ROCKET (ARUGULA) INSTEAD OF ICEBERG LETTUCE.

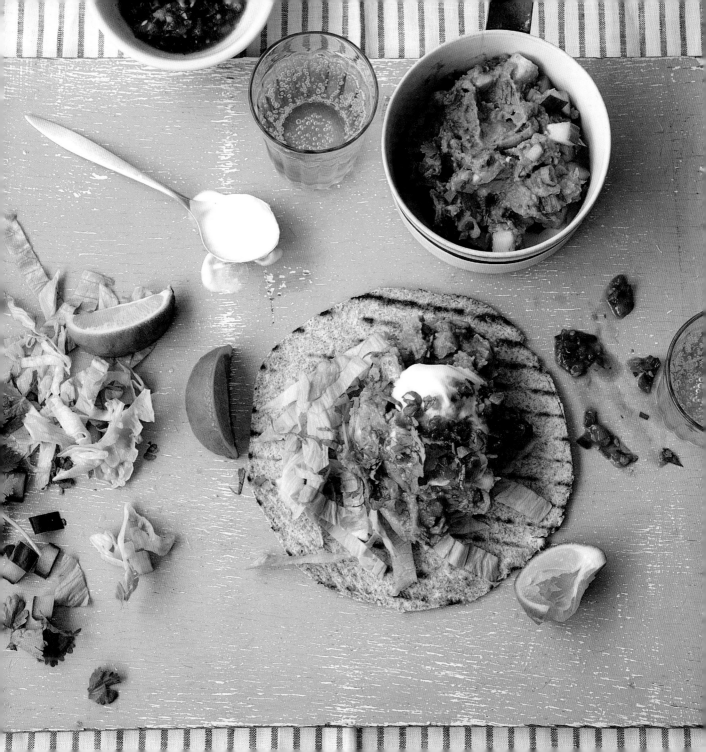

# MOZZARELLA CHICKEN PARCELS

Per serving
200 kcals
Fat: 5.5g
Fibre: 3g
Low GI

**This is an easy way to cook chicken, and the sun-dried tomato and mozzarella filling keeps it juicy and succulent. In summer, you can cook the foil parcels over the hot coals on a barbecue. Check that they are thoroughly cooked all the way through before removing them – chicken must always be well cooked.**

spray olive oil

2 x 100g/3½oz skinless, boneless chicken breasts

1 sun-dried tomato, drained and thinly sliced

4 fresh basil leaves, torn

50g/1¾oz reduced-fat mozzarella cheese, diced

grated zest and juice of 1 lemon

freshly ground black pepper

1 small yellow (bell) pepper, deseeded and cut into chunks

1 small red onion, cut into wedges

1 courgette (zucchini), cut into chunks

fresh thyme, oregano or rosemary sprigs

Serves 2
Prep: 15 minutes
Cook: 25 minutes

Preheat the oven to 200°C/400°F/Gas mark 6. Lightly spray two large squares of foil with oil.

Make a deep slit in each chicken breast with a sharp knife and open it up to create a pocket. Fill the pocket with the sun-dried tomato, basil and mozzarella. Place a chicken breast on each square of foil.

Sprinkle the lemon zest and juice over the chicken, together with some black pepper.

Draw the foil from the corners up into the centre to completely enclose the chicken and seal the parcels so the chicken is loosely wrapped. Bake in the oven for about 25 minutes, or until the chicken is thoroughly cooked and the mozzarella has melted.

Meanwhile, put the prepared vegetables into an ovenproof dish or roasting tin. Add the herbs and season with pepper. Spray lightly with oil and roast with the chicken for 25 minutes, or until tender and slightly charred.

SLIM FACT...
REDUCED-FAT MOZZARELLA HAS HALF THE FAT OF THE REGULAR SORT AND FEWER CALORIES: 184 CALORIES AND 10.2G FAT PER 100G/3½OZ AS OPPOSED TO 275 CALORIES AND 20.6G FAT.

# LEMON
# CHICKEN KEBABS

**You can use metal, bamboo or wooden kebab skewers for the chicken. If using wooden or bamboo ones, soak them first in water to prevent them burning under the hot grill or over the hot coals of the barbecue.**

300g/10½oz skinless chicken breast
fillets, cut into chunks
juice of 1 lemon
good pinch of crushed fennel seeds
2 garlic cloves, crushed
freshly ground black pepper
spray oil
few fresh parsley sprigs, chopped
lemon wedges, to serve

**For the warm rocket and
mushroom salad**
spray oil
150g/5½oz button (white)
mushrooms, sliced
100g/3½oz wild rocket (arugula)
few drops of balsamic vinegar

Serves 2
Prep: 10 minutes
Marinate: 30 minutes
Cook: 10–15 minutes

Place the chicken in a bowl with the lemon juice. Add the fennel seeds, garlic and black pepper. Stir well to coat the chicken, then cover the bowl and marinate in the refrigerator for 30 minutes.

Preheat the grill (broiler) or barbecue. Thread the marinated chicken onto some kebab skewers and spray lightly with oil. Lay them in a foil-lined grill pan and cook under the hot grill or place over hot coals for about 10–15 minutes, turning the kebabs occasionally, until the chicken is cooked through and golden brown.

While the chicken is cooking, make the salad: lightly spray a small frying pan with oil and place over a medium heat. When it's hot, add the mushrooms and cook, turning them occasionally, until tender and golden brown.

Toss the hot mushrooms with the rocket. Divide between two serving plates and drizzle with balsamic vinegar. Place the chicken kebabs on top. Sprinkle with chopped parsley and squeeze the lemon wedges over the top. Serve immediately.

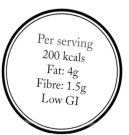

Per serving
200 kcals
Fat: 4g
Fibre: 1.5g
Low GI

# MEXICAN BEEF SALSA POT

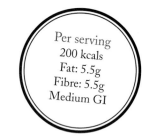

Per serving
200 kcals
Fat: 5.5g
Fibre: 5.5g
Medium GI

**In this delicious variation on a traditional chilli con carne, the hot salsa is stirred into the stew. Check the labels carefully when buying ready-made salsa – different brands vary enormously in their calorie and fat content, so look for the lowest available.**

spray oil
1 small red onion, chopped
1 small red (bell) pepper, deseeded and chopped
200g/7oz lean minced (ground) beef (max 5% fat)
1 tsp chilli powder
1 x 200g/7oz can chopped tomatoes
100ml/3½fl oz/scant ½ cup beef stock
100g/3½oz canned kidney beans, rinsed and drained
50g/1¾oz reduced-fat hot salsa
freshly ground black pepper
few fresh coriander (cilantro) sprigs, chopped
2 tbsp virtually fat-free fromage frais

Serves 2
Prep: 15 minutes
Cook: 30–35 minutes

Lightly spray a large pan with oil and place over a medium heat. Add the onion and red pepper and cook for 5 minutes until starting to soften. Add the beef and cook, stirring, for 2–3 minutes until browned.

Stir in the chilli powder, tomatoes and stock and bring to the boil. Reduce the heat, add the kidney beans and simmer gently for 20 minutes, or until the beef is cooked. Stir in the salsa and season to taste with pepper.

Ladle into bowls and serve immediately sprinkled with chopped coriander and topped with a dollop of fromage frais.

OR TRY THIS…
THIS BECOMES A VERY SATISFYING 300-CALORIE SUPPER IF YOU SERVE EACH PORTION WITH 75G/2¾OZ/SCANT ½ CUP BOILED BROWN RICE (30G/1OZ/SCANT ¼ CUP DRY WEIGHT).

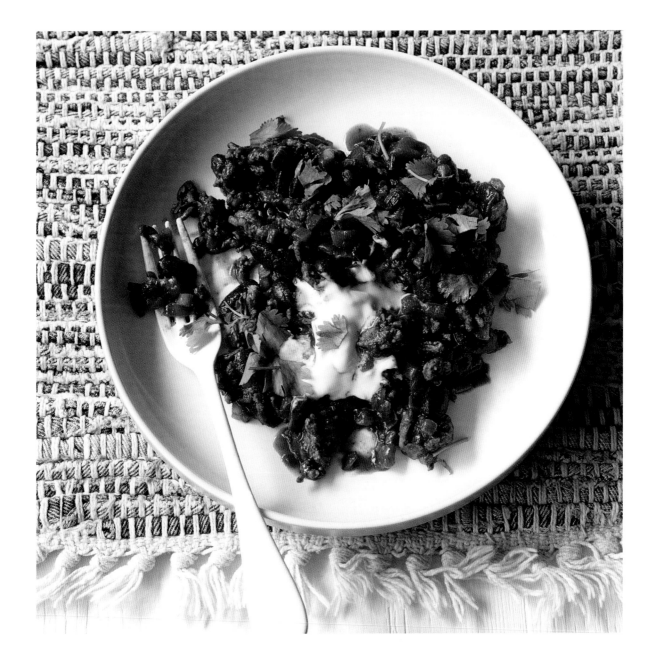

# SPANISH SUMMER BAKE

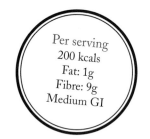

**This is a meal in itself, or you can serve it with grilled chicken or fish. It will serve four people as a side dish, and if you give everyone a 90g/3¼oz grilled chicken breast fillet or a 100g/3½oz grilled white fish fillet (skinned and boned), you will still end up with a 200-calorie meal.**

1 red (bell) pepper, deseeded and cut into chunks
1 small aubergine (eggplant), sliced
1 small red onion, thinly sliced
spray olive oil
300g/10½oz potatoes, peeled and thinly sliced
salt and freshly ground black pepper
few fresh parsley sprigs, chopped

For the tomato sauce
spray olive oil
1 onion, finely chopped
2 garlic cloves, crushed
1 x 200g/7oz can chopped tomatoes
few fresh basil sprigs, chopped
salt and freshly ground black pepper
few drops of balsamic vinegar

Serves 2
Prep: 15 minutes
Cook: 55 minutes

Preheat the oven to 200°C/400°F/Gas mark 6.

To make the tomato sauce, lightly spray a large non-stick frying pan with oil and place over a low heat. Add the onion and garlic and cook for at least 5 minutes until softened and golden.

Add the tomatoes and basil and turn up the heat. Cook for 8–10 minutes until the sauce is thickened and reduced. Season to taste with salt and pepper and add the balsamic vinegar.

While the sauce is cooking, put the red pepper, aubergine and red onion in a roasting tin. Spray with a little oil and roast in the oven for about 10 minutes.

Arrange a layer of sliced potatoes in a shallow ovenproof dish. Cover with a layer of roasted vegetables and then a layer of tomato sauce. Continue layering up in this way, finishing with a layer of potatoes and a drizzle of tomato sauce.

Cover the dish with foil and bake in the oven for 20 minutes, then remove the foil and bake for a further 15–20 minutes, or until the vegetables are tender and the top is crisp and golden brown. Sprinkle with chopped parsley and serve immediately.

# CRUNCHY VEGETABLE CROQUETTES

**This is a delicious way of using up leftover vegetables, as long as they are not starchy (potatoes, parsnips, sweet potatoes). The white sauce has to be very thick to bind the vegetables inside the crisp coating of the croquettes.**

175g/6oz cooked vegetables, such as peas, diced carrot, cabbage, spring greens, broccoli, cauliflower, (bell) peppers, courgette (zucchini), mushrooms
few fresh parsley sprigs, finely chopped
½ small egg, beaten
15g/½oz/generous ¼ cup fresh breadcrumbs
spray oil
1 large head red chicory or radicchio
1 red apple, cored and thinly sliced
¼ red onion, chopped
few fresh chives, snipped
1 tbsp oil-free vinaigrette dressing
2 tsp cranberry sauce, to serve

**For the white sauce**
1 tbsp cornflour (cornstarch)
150ml/¼ pint/⅔ cup skimmed (lowfat) milk
50g/1¾oz/scant ¼ cup virtually fat-free natural fromage frais
good pinch of ground nutmeg
salt and freshly ground black pepper

Serves 2
Prep: 15 minutes
Chill: 30 minutes
Cook: 10 minutes

Make the white sauce: mix the cornflour with a little of the milk until it is a smooth paste. Heat the remaining milk in a saucepan and when it starts to boil, stir in the cornflour mixture. Reduce the heat to a simmer and cook, stirring, for 2 minutes until the sauce is very thick and smooth. Remove from the heat and beat in the fromage frais, nutmeg and seasoning.

Stir the cooked vegetables and parsley into the sauce and leave to cool. The mixture should be quite firm.

Divide the mixture into four portions and shape into croquettes with your hands. Dip them in the beaten egg and then roll in the breadcrumbs. Cover and chill in the refrigerator for at least 30 minutes to firm them up.

Lightly spray a non-stick frying pan with oil and place over a medium heat. When the pan is hot, add the croquettes and cook for about 5 minutes, turning them occasionally, until crisp and golden brown all over.

Meanwhile, mix the chicory, apple, onion and chives together in a bowl. Add the vinaigrette dressing and toss everything lightly together. Serve the hot croquettes and salad with the cranberry sauce.

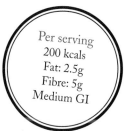

Per serving
200 kcals
Fat: 2.5g
Fibre: 5g
Medium GI

# GRILLED VEGETABLE AND HALLOUMI STACKS

**Vegetable stacks are healthy, low-calorie and simple to assemble and cook. If you don't like aubergine, use a large beefsteak tomato, cut into thick slices, instead. Halloumi cheese is very filling and keeps its shape when it's cooked rather than melting, making it ideal for veggie stacks and kebabs.**

2 large Portobello or field mushrooms
spray olive oil
1 small aubergine (eggplant), cut horizontally into thick slices
1 x 200g/7oz butternut squash, peeled, deseeded and cut into thick horizontal slices
2 courgettes (zucchini), cut into long diagonal slices
salt and freshly ground black pepper
60g/2¼oz reduced-fat halloumi cheese, sliced
50g/1¾oz baby spinach leaves
2 tsp oil-free vinaigrette dressing
balsamic vinegar, for drizzling
few fresh basil leaves, shredded
1 tbsp reduced-fat green pesto

Serves 2
Prep: 15 minutes
Cook: 20–25 minutes

Remove and discard the stalks from the mushrooms, then spray the mushrooms lightly with oil. Spray the aubergine, butternut squash and courgettes lightly with oil.

Place a non-stick ridged griddle pan over a medium heat. When it's hot, cook the prepared vegetables in batches, a few at a time, until they are tender and slightly charred. Season lightly with salt and freshly ground black pepper and keep warm.

Grill the halloumi for 2–3 minutes on each side, or until golden brown.

Toss the spinach in the vinaigrette dressing and divide between two serving plates. Assemble a vegetable and halloumi stack in the centre of each plate, beginning with the mushrooms at the base. Drizzle with balsamic vinegar, scatter over the basil and serve immediately with the pesto.

SLIM FACT...
REDUCED-FAT PESTO AVERAGES OUT AT 20 CALORIES PER TEASPOON – LESS THAN ONE-QUARTER OF THE CALORIES AND FAT OF REGULAR PESTO. AS IT HAS A STRONG, DISTINCTIVE FLAVOUR, A LITTLE GOES A LONG WAY. STIR A TEASPOONFUL INTO YOGURT OR VIRTUALLY FAT-FREE FROMAGE FRAIS AS A DIP OR SAUCE FOR GRILLED MEAT, CHICKEN OR PRAWNS (SHRIMP).

Per serving
200 kcals
Fat: 8g
Fibre: 6.5g
Low GI

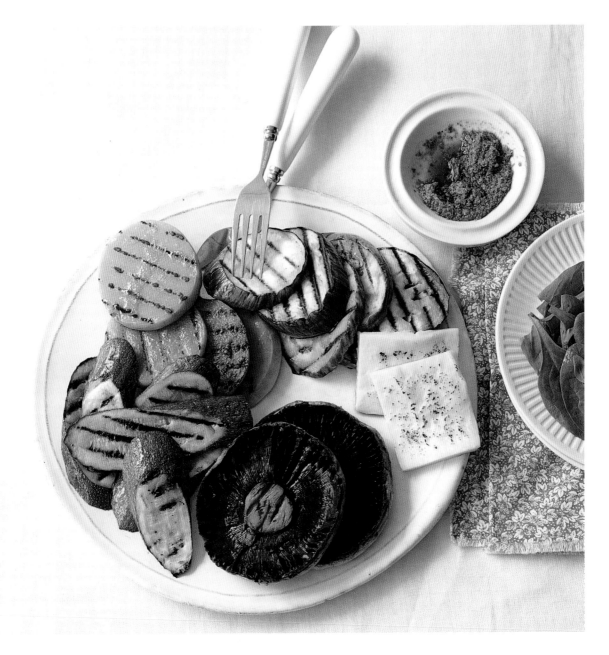

# THAI
# PRAWN SKEWERS

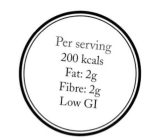

Per serving
200 kcals
Fat: 2g
Fibre: 2g
Low GI

**Prawns (shrimp) are great when you're watching your weight, as they are low in calories and fat. Raw prawns have only 70 calories and 0.7g fat per 100g/3½oz – much lower than white and oily fish or even chicken. And they're so simple and quick to cook, too.**

300g/10½oz raw tiger prawns (jumbo shrimp), peeled
60g/2¼oz/scant ⅔ cup bean sprouts
¼ small cucumber, cut into matchstick strips
1 yellow (bell) pepper, deseeded and thinly sliced
3 spring onions (scallions), chopped
2 tbsp chopped fresh coriander (cilantro)

**For the marinade and dressing**
1 hot red chilli, finely chopped
1 tsp grated fresh root ginger
1 garlic clove, crushed
1 tbsp nam pla (Thai fish sauce)
1 tbsp light soy sauce
juice of 1 lime
artificial sweetener, to taste

Serves 2
Prep: 15 minutes
Cook: 4–6 minutes

Preheat the grill (broiler). Soak two or four wooden or bamboo skewers in water to stop them burning under the hot grill. Mix all the marinade ingredients together in a small bowl.

Thread the prawns onto the skewers, arrange them on a foil-lined grill pan and brush lightly with some of the marinade.

Cook the prawn skewers under the hot grill for about 4–6 minutes, turning them halfway through, until they turn pink all over. Don't overcook, or they will become dry – they should be juicy and succulent.

In a bowl, combine the bean sprouts, cucumber, yellow pepper, spring onions and coriander. Add the remaining marinade and toss to lightly coat everything. Serve the hot prawn skewers with the salad.

OR TRY THIS...
SUBSTITUTE 200G/7OZ SKINNED CHICKEN BREAST FILLETS FOR THE PRAWNS; MARINATE AND COOK IN THE SAME WAY. THE CALORIE COUNT REMAINS THE SAME.

# GRILLED COD AND LENTILS

**Fish and lentils might seem an unusual combination, but they complement each other very well: the succulent flaky texture of the cod with the earthy flavour of the Puy lentils. If you can't buy these, you can substitute green or brown Continental ones, but not the split red or yellow ones which turn to mush when cooked.**

50g/1¾oz/¼ cup Puy lentils
50g/1¾oz/¼ cup diced carrot
1 celery stick, chopped
1 tsp oil-free vinaigrette dressing
2 tbsp chopped fresh parsley
freshly ground black pepper
2 x 100g/3½oz cod steaks or fillets, skinned and boned
200g/7oz courgettes (zucchini)
squeeze of lemon juice

Serves 2
Prep: 10 minutes
Cook: 25 minutes

Per serving
200 kcals
Fat: 2.5g
Fibre: 5g
Low GI

Put the lentils in a saucepan with the carrot and celery and cover with cold water. Bring to the boil, then reduce the heat and cover with a lid. Simmer gently for 20 minutes, or until the lentils and vegetables are cooked and tender.

Drain well and stir the vinaigrette and chopped parsley into the lentil and vegetable mixture. Season to taste with pepper.

While the lentils are cooking, preheat the grill (broiler) to high, or the oven to 180°C/350°F/Gas mark 4. Grill the cod for 3–4 minutes on each side until cooked right through. Or wrap them in foil and bake in the oven for about 15 minutes.

Using a potato peeler, thinly slice the courgettes lengthways into long ribbons. Cook in boiling water or steam them for 2 minutes until just tender but not mushy – they must keep their shape and lovely fresh green colour.

Divide the warm lentil mixture between two serving plates and place the cod on top. Squeeze over a little lemon juice and serve with the courgette ribbons, seasoned with black pepper.

OR TRY THIS…
STIR A DASH OF BALSAMIC VINEGAR AND ½ TEASPOON DIJON MUSTARD INTO THE VINAIGRETTE FOR A MORE PIQUANT FLAVOUR. THIS ADDS ONLY 2 CALORIES PER SERVING.

# PAN-SEARED COD WITH BUTTER BEANS

**Here's a quick and easy supper for when you come in from work. You can use fresh or frozen cod, or haddock or monkfish (angler fish) – any firm-fleshed white fish will work well.**

spray oil
1 onion, finely chopped
2 garlic cloves, crushed
1 tbsp balsamic vinegar
225g/8oz cherry tomatoes, halved
200g/7oz canned butter (lima) beans, drained
salt and freshly ground black pepper
2 x 125g/4½oz thick cod fillets, skinned
squeeze of lemon juice
2 tbsp chopped fresh parsley

Serves 2
Prep: 5 minutes
Cook: 15 minutes

Lightly spray a frying pan with oil and place over a low heat. Add the onion and garlic and cook gently for about 5 minutes, or until softened.

Stir in the balsamic vinegar and cherry tomatoes and continue cooking for 5 minutes. Add the butter beans and cook gently for a further 5 minutes. Season to taste with salt and pepper.

Meanwhile, spray a non-stick frying pan with oil and place over a medium heat. When hot, add the cod fillets and cook for 4–5 minutes on each side, or until cooked right through.

Divide the tomato and bean mixture between two serving plates and place the cod on top. Add a good squeeze of lemon juice and a sprinkling of parsley.

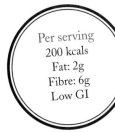

Per serving
200 kcals
Fat: 2g
Fibre: 6g
Low GI

OR TRY THIS...
IF YOU DON'T HAVE CANNED BUTTER BEANS, USE HARICOT OR CANNELLINI BEANS INSTEAD. ALWAYS RINSE CANNED BEANS WELL BEFORE DRAINING AND USING IN COOKED DISHES OR SALADS.

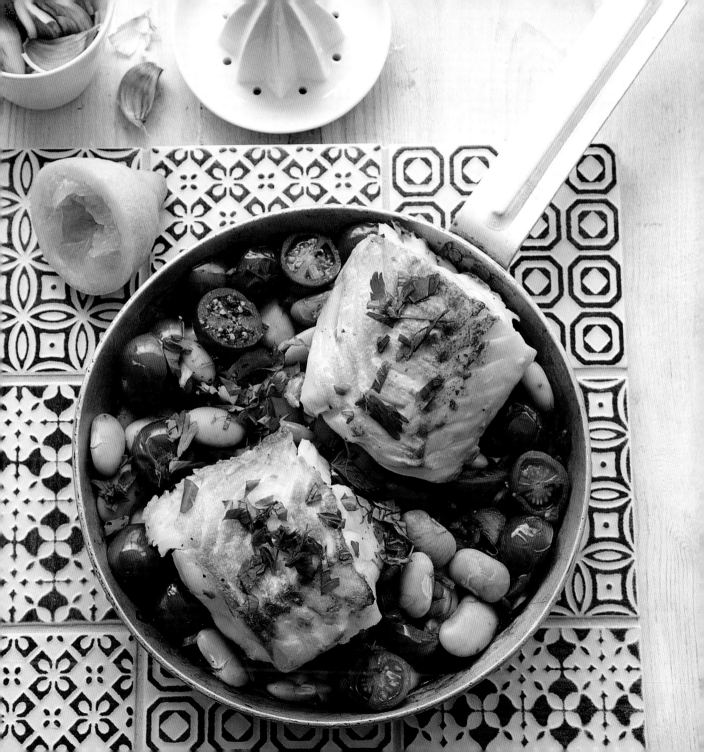

# THAI PRAWN AND AUBERGINE CURRY

**Thai curry pastes vary considerably in their heat, so add 1 tablespoon and taste before adding more; if you don't like hot curry, you may not need to add 2 tablespoons. Remember that you can always add more heat to a curry, but it's difficult to tone it down and make it milder. For a Thai red curry, substitute red curry paste.**

spray oil

2 shallots, thinly sliced

2.5cm/1in piece fresh root ginger, peeled and chopped

1 small aubergine (eggplant), thinly sliced

2 tbsp Thai green curry paste

150g/5½oz cherry tomatoes, halved

150ml/¼ pint/⅔ cup reduced-fat coconut milk

1 tsp nam pla (Thai fish sauce)

175g/6oz peeled raw tiger prawns (jumbo shrimp)

few fresh coriander (cilantro) sprigs, chopped

few basil leaves, shredded

Serves 2

Prep: 10 minutes

Cook: 20 minutes

Spray a non-stick frying pan lightly with oil and place over a medium heat. Add the shallots and ginger and cook for 5 minutes. When they are golden and translucent, add the aubergine and cook gently for 4–5 minutes until tender and golden brown on both sides.

Stir in the curry paste and cook for 1 minute, then add the tomatoes and cook for a further 2 minutes. Pour in the coconut milk and nam pla and heat through gently.

Add the prawns and cook, turning them over once or twice, for 2–3 minutes until they turn pink on both sides. Sprinkle with coriander and basil, and serve.

SLIM FACT...
IF YOU SERVE A CURRY WITH PLAIN BOILED RICE, YOU WILL ADD 100 CALORIES AND 0.5G FAT FOR EACH 30G/1OZ/ SCANT ¼ CUP DRY WEIGHT OR 75G/2¾OZ/SCANT ½ CUP COOKED WEIGHT.

Per serving
200 kcals
Fat: 9.5g
Fibre: 5g
Low GI

# MARYLAND CRABCAKES

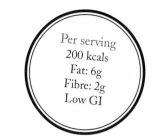

Per serving
200 kcals
Fat: 6g
Fibre: 2g
Low GI

**These crabcakes can be prepared several hours in advance and then chilled in the refrigerator until you are ready to cook them. If you can't get fresh white crabmeat, you can buy it frozen or you could use canned.**

1 small free-range egg, beaten
2 tbsp extra-light mayonnaise
¼ teaspoon Dijon mustard
grated zest and juice of ½ lemon
2 tbsp chopped fresh parsley
or tarragon
300g/10½oz white crabmeat
(fresh or frozen)
salt and freshly ground black pepper
plain (all-purpose) flour, for dusting
spray oil
2 tsp sweet chilli sauce (optional)

**For the tomato and basil salad**
2 large ripe tomatoes, thinly sliced
½ small red onion, finely chopped
few fresh basil leaves, torn into strips
good-quality balsamic vinegar,
for drizzling

Serves 2
Prep: 15 minutes
Chill: 1 hour
Cook: 8 minutes

In a bowl, mix together the beaten egg, mayonnaise and mustard until well combined. Add the lemon zest and juice, chopped herbs and crabmeat. Season lightly with salt and pepper.

Shape the mixture with your hands into four patties. Wrap in clingfilm (plastic wrap) and chill in the refrigerator for at least 1 hour to firm up.

Dust the chilled crabcakes lightly with flour. Lightly spray a non-stick frying pan with oil and place over a medium heat. Add the crabcakes to the hot pan and cook for about 4 minutes on each side until golden brown and crisp.

Meanwhile, arrange the tomatoes, onion and basil on two serving plates. Season with salt and pepper and drizzle with balsamic vinegar. Serve with the hot crabcakes and a little sweet chilli dipping sauce, if wished.

OR TRY THIS...
FOR SPICIER CRAB CAKES, ADD A DASH OF TABASCO SAUCE TO THE MIXTURE BEFORE SHAPING IT INTO PATTIES – NOT TOO MUCH, AS IT IS VERY HOT.

# SMOKED SALMON FISHCAKES

**Smoked salmon is an oily fish and high in fat, but it's the healthy Omega-3 sort, which is good for your heart. You need only a little salmon to flavour these fishcakes, providing 45 calories and 2.5g fat per serving.**

200g/7oz potatoes, peeled and diced
50g/1¾oz smoked salmon trimmings, roughly chopped
1 tbsp chopped capers
2 spring onions (scallions), finely chopped
1 red chilli, deseeded and finely chopped
few fresh dill sprigs, finely chopped
few fresh chives, snipped
salt and freshly ground black pepper
grated zest and juice of ½ lime
½ beaten egg
plain (all-purpose) flour, for dusting
spray oil

**For the garlic and lime mayonnaise**
2 tbsp extra-light mayonnaise
1 garlic clove, crushed
grated zest and juice of ½ lime

**To serve**
salad leaves
100g/3½oz cherry tomatoes, halved
2 tsp oil-free vinaigrette dressing

Serves 2
Prep: 15 minutes
Chill: at least 1 hour
Cook: 20 minutes

Cook the potatoes in a saucepan of lightly salted boiling water for 10–12 minutes until cooked and tender. Drain in a colander and leave to cool.

Mash the potatoes, removing any lumps. Put the mashed potato in a bowl with the smoked salmon, capers, spring onions, chilli, herbs, salt and pepper, lime zest and juice, and the beaten egg and mix well together.

Divide the mixture in half and, using your hands, shape each portion into a fishcake. Dust lightly with flour, then cover and chill in the refrigerator until you are ready to cook the fishcakes.

Combine all the ingredients for the garlic and lime mayonnaise in a small bowl.

Spray a non-stick frying pan lightly with oil and cook the fishcakes over a medium heat for 4–5 minutes on each side until they are piping hot and golden brown.

Serve immediately with the garlic and lime mayonnaise, salad leaves and cherry tomatoes tossed in the oil-free vinaigrette.

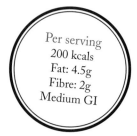

Per serving
200 kcals
Fat: 4.5g
Fibre: 2g
Medium GI

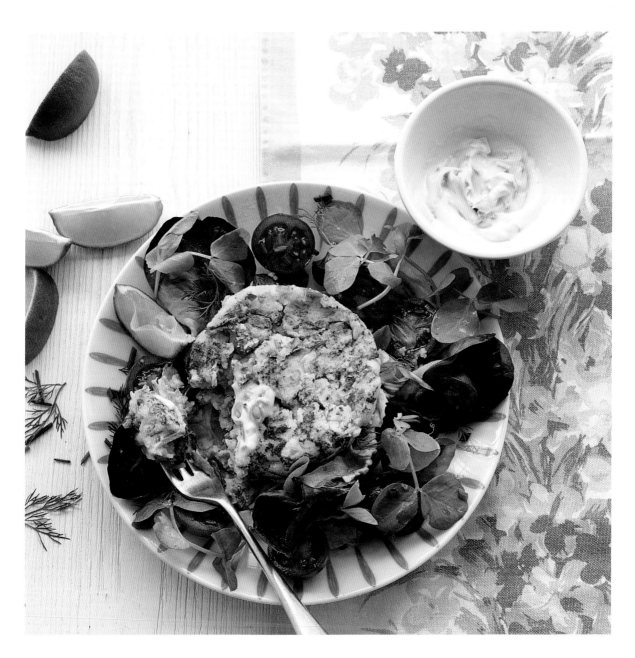

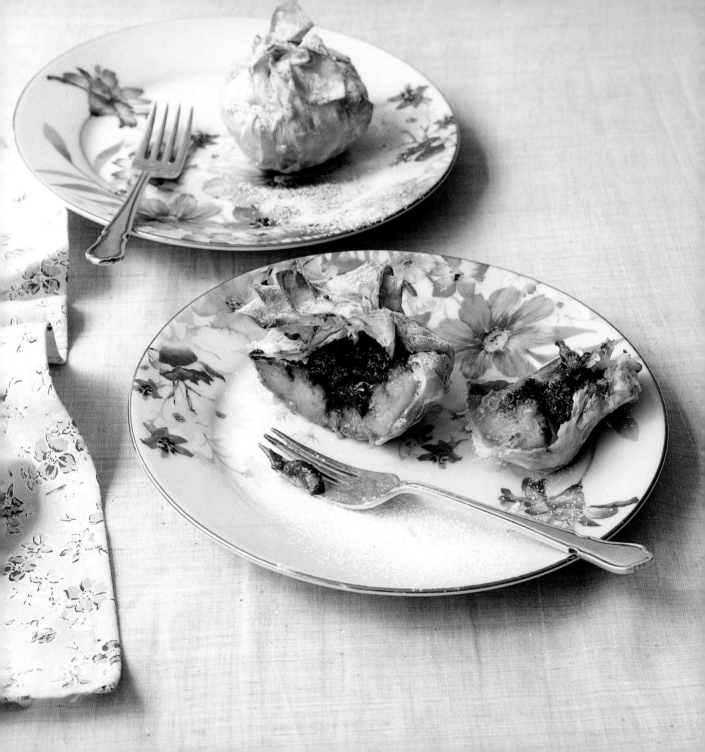

# CHOCOLATE FRUITY FILO PARCELS

Even when you're watching what you eat, you're still allowed the occasional sweet treat. These fruity filo parcels will appeal to chocoholics and at 200 calories each you can plan for them within your daily calorie intake. Different brands of filo pastry come in varying sizes. I used sheets cut down to 15cm/6in squares. You can always freeze any unused sheets for another occasion.

4 x 15g/½oz sheets filo pastry (dough)
1 small egg, beaten
4 amaretti biscuits (cookies), crushed
60g/2¼oz dark (semisweet) chocolate, grated
2 tbsp very low-fat natural fromage frais
2 ripe peaches, halved, peeled and stoned
icing (confectioners') sugar, for dusting

Serves 4
Prep: 15 minutes
Cook: 10–15 minutesPerspero in con conemquam quist inis erspictur

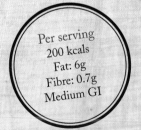

Per serving
200 kcals
Fat: 6g
Fibre: 0.7g
Medium GI

Preheat the oven to 200°C/400°F/Gas mark 6 and line a baking tray with baking parchment.

Lightly brush each sheet of filo pastry with beaten egg, then fold in half widthways and brush again with beaten egg.

In a small bowl, mix together the amaretti biscuits, chocolate and fromage frais, then using a teaspoon, fill the peach halves with the mixture.

Place a filled peach half in the centre of each filo pastry sheet and bring up the corners to meet at the top in the middle. Pinch the tops together with your fingers to seal them and to make an attractive 'crown' shape.

Brush the filo parcels with the remaining beaten egg and place them on the prepared baking tray. Bake in the oven for 10–15 minutes until the pastry is crisp and golden. Dust lightly with icing sugar and serve hot.

OR TRY THIS…
USE NECTARINES OR FRESH APRICOTS INSTEAD OF PEACHES. IF YOU SERVE THEM WITH 0% FAT GREEK YOGURT, A TABLESPOONFUL ON THE SIDE OF EACH FILO PARCEL WILL ADD 9 CALORIES.

# SUMMER FRUIT MINI PAVLOVAS

**You can buy ready-made meringue nests in most supermarkets, which takes all the hard work out of this dessert. Store any unused meringues in an airtight container for up to 1 month. If you prefer the flavour of dark bitter chocolate, use this instead of the sweeter white variety.**

100g/3½oz/scant ½ cup 0% fat Greek yogurt

2 x 13g/½oz meringue nests

200g/7oz/1⅓ cups mixed summer fruits, such as strawberries, raspberries, blueberries, redcurrants, chopped peaches, pitted cherries

icing (confectioners') sugar, for dusting

30g/1oz white chocolate, broken into pieces

Serves 2
Prep: 10 minutes
Cook: 5 minutes

Swirl the yogurt into the centre and on the top of each meringue nest, then put each meringue on a serving plate.

Top with the summer fruits and scatter any leftover fruit around the plate. Dust lightly with icing sugar.

Melt the white chocolate by placing it in a heatproof bowl set over a small pan of gently simmering water.

Drizzle the melted chocolate over the fruit and serve.

Per serving
200 kcals
Fat: 4.5g
Fibre: 1.5g
Low GI

OR TRY THIS...
IN THE WINTER, SUBSTITUTE SLICED KIWI FRUIT, FRESH POMEGRANATE SEEDS OR CLEMENTINE SEGMENTS FOR THE SUMMER FRUITS. VIRTUALLY FAT-FREE NATURAL FROMAGE FRAIS CAN BE USED INSTEAD OF THE GREEK YOGURT. THE CALORIE AND FAT CONTENT ARE THE SAME.

# TIRAMISU

We've used Quark, a really low-calorie soft cheese, in this recipe because it is so low in fat and has a great texture. Most good supermarkets sell it, but if you can't find it you can substitute virtually fat-free natural fromage frais, which has the same fat content but even fewer calories.

1 egg yolk

1 tbsp caster (superfine) sugar

1–2 drops vanilla extract

200g/7oz/scant 1 cup Quark soft cheese

60ml/2fl oz/¼ cup hot strong espresso coffee

1 tsp Tia Maria

8 sponge (lady) fingers

½ tsp unsweetened cocoa powder, sifted

Serves 2

Prep: 15 minutes

In a bowl, beat the egg yolk and sugar with a wooden spoon until thick and creamy. Stir in the vanilla and beat in the Quark.

Pour the hot espresso into another bowl and stir in the Tia Maria. Dip four of the sponge fingers into this and place them in the bottom of two small glass dishes or sundae glasses. Cover with half of the creamy cheese mixture.

Dip the remaining sponge fingers into the coffee and arrange on top of the Quark. Spoon the rest of the Quark on top, then smooth the surface and dust lightly with sifted cocoa. Chill in the refrigerator until required.

Per serving
200 kcals
Fat: 2.2g
Fibre: trace
Medium GI

NOTE:
THIS TIRAMISU IS MADE WITH A RAW EGG YOLK, SO IF YOU ARE PREGNANT, BREASTFEEDING, ELDERLY OR ARE UNWELL IT'S ADVISABLE TO AVOID EATING RAW EGG.

# APPLE AND BLACKBERRY STRUDEL

**Strudel is easier to make than you might think and this version includes ground almonds, which give it a delicious flavour and moistness. When blackberries and apples are plentiful in the autumn, it's a good idea to cook them in batches and freeze them to use in strudels, pies and crumbles. Different brands of filo pastry come in varying sizes. I used sheets cut down to 15cm/6in square. You can always freeze any unused sheets for another occasion.**

675g/1½lb dessert apples, such as Granny Smith, Cox, peeled, cored and diced
175g/6oz/1¼ cups blackberries
25g/1oz/generous ¼ cup ground almonds
grated zest of 1 lemon
25g/1oz/2 tbsp granulated sugar substitute
6 x 15g/½oz sheets filo pastry (dough)
spray oil
icing (confectioners') sugar, for dusting
6 tbsp 0% fat Greek yogurt, to serve

Serves 6
Prep: 15 minutes
Cook: 30–35 minutes

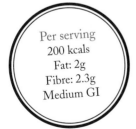

Per serving
200 kcals
Fat: 2g
Fibre: 2.3g
Medium GI

Preheat the oven to 190°C/375°F/Gas mark 5.

Mix the apples, berries, ground almonds, lemon zest and sugar together in a bowl.

Spread a sheet of filo pastry out on a clean board or work surface and spray lightly with oil. Place the remaining sheets on top, spraying each one with oil.

Spoon the apple and blackberry mixture lengthways along the centre of the filo pastry, in a long strip, not quite reaching the edge of the pastry at each end. Fold the ends of the pastry in over the filling and then fold one of the long sides over the filling, tucking it in neatly underneath the filling. Spray the pastry lightly with oil and then cover with the remaining pastry to make a sealed long parcel.

Lift the strudel, seam-side down, onto a non-stick baking sheet and bake in the oven for 30–35 minutes until crisp and golden. Check after 20 minutes and if the pastry seems to be browning too much, cover it loosely with foil.

Leave to cool a little before dusting the strudel with icing sugar and cutting into slices. Serve each slice with a dollop of Greek yogurt.

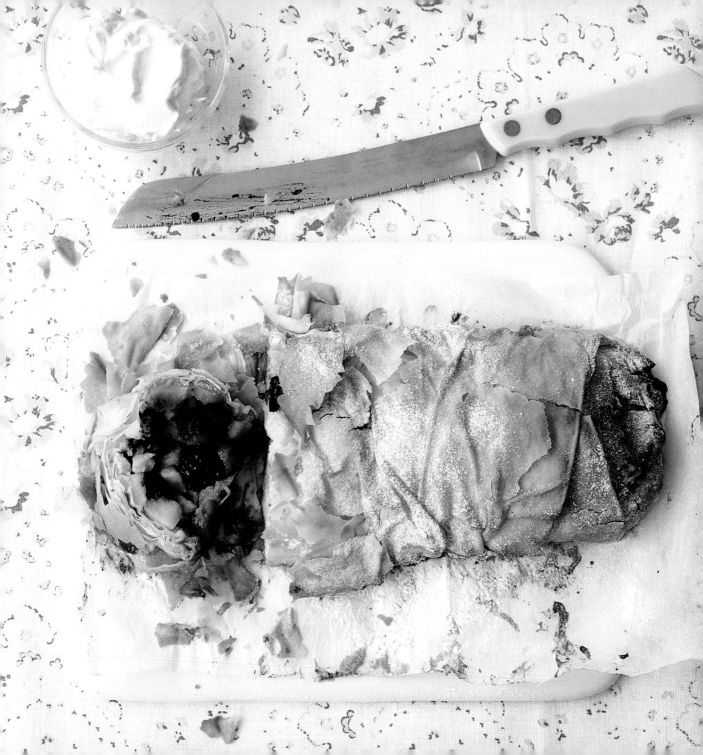

# BAILEYS BANOFFEE CUSTARD

**If you are a fan of banoffee pie, which is laden with sugar and fat, here's a delicious low-calorie alternative that won't affect your waistline. The 0% fat Greek yogurt is better than other very low-fat varieties because it has such a firm and creamy texture.**

2 tsp muscovado sugar

2 tsp custard powder

125ml/4fl oz/½ cup skimmed (lowfat) milk

1 tbsp Bailey's Original Irish Cream Liqueur

150g/5½oz/⅔ cup 0% fat Greek yogurt

1 ripe medium banana, mashed

1 egg white

unsweetened cocoa powder, sifted, for dusting

Serves 2

Prep: 15 minutes

Mix the muscovado sugar and custard powder together with a little of the milk until you have a smooth mixture that's free of lumps.

Heat the remaining milk with the Bailey's in a small saucepan. As soon as it starts to boil, remove from the heat and pour the milk on to the custard mixture, stirring well.

Pour the custard back into the warm pan and place over a low heat, stirring all the time with a wooden spoon until the custard thickens. When you have a smooth custard, remove from the heat and leave until it's completely cold.

Fold the yogurt and mashed banana into the cold custard.

Whisk the egg white in a clean, dry bowl until it's really stiff, then using a metal spoon, fold it gently into the custard, distributing it evenly.

Divide the custard between two tall glasses or glass dishes and dust lightly with sifted cocoa. Serve or chill in the refrigerator until required.

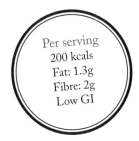

Per serving
200 kcals
Fat: 1.3g
Fibre: 2g
Low GI

# NO-COOK CAKE

**You can enjoy a slice of this on its own straight from the refrigerator or serve it as a dessert with a dollop of virtually fat-free fromage frais and some fresh strawberries or raspberries. It will keep for several days in the refrigerator, but make it only when you are expecting guests so that you are not tempted to go back for 'just a little bit more'. It's good to treat yourself occasionally, but cakes and desserts should not be part of your everyday diet.**

125g/4oz dark (semisweet) chocolate (70% minimum cocoa solids), broken into squares
60g/2¼oz/¼cup low-fat margarine
1 egg white
125g/4½oz gingernut biscuits (cookies)
100g/3½oz/½ cup ready-to-eat dried apricots, chopped
30g/1oz/¼ cup dried cranberries

Makes 8 slices
Prep: 15 minutes
Chill: 2–3 hours

Put the chocolate into a heatproof basin with the margarine. Set it over a saucepan of simmering water and stir gently until combined and melted. Remove from the heat.

Beat the egg white in a clean, dry bowl until it forms stiff peaks. With a metal spoon, fold it gently into the melted chocolate mixture, using a figure of eight motion, and mix thoroughly to distribute the egg white evenly.

Roughly crush the biscuits with a rolling pin to leave some chunky pieces as well as crumbs. Stir them into the chocolate mixture with the apricots and cranberries.

Spoon the mixture into an 18cm/7in cake tin and spread it out evenly, smoothing the top. Chill in the refrigerator for 2–3 hours, or until firm. Serve cut into slices.

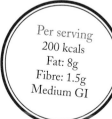

Per serving
200 kcals
Fat: 8g
Fibre: 1.5g
Medium GI

SLIM FACT...
YOU CAN SUBSTITUTE LOW-FAT DIGESTIVE BISCUITS
(GRAHAM CRACKERS) FOR THE GINGERNUTS BUT,
SURPRISINGLY, THEY ARE HIGHER IN CALORIES AND FAT.

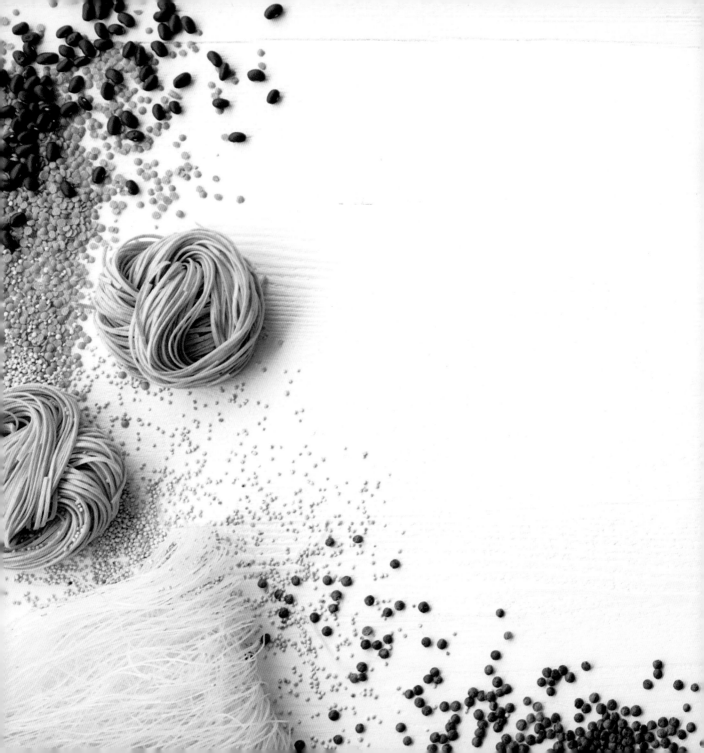

# 300 calories

# PORRIDGE WITH FRUIT COMPÔTE

**Oats are not only really healthy and packed with essential nutrients but they also have a low GI rating and are great for promoting weight loss. They are the perfect breakfast food because they reduce hunger pangs and make us feel fuller for longer, so we are less likely to be tempted to snack mid-morning. Don't sweeten your porridge with sugar or syrup – this fruit compôte makes a great alternative topping.**

85g/3oz/1 cup jumbo rolled oats
pinch of salt
200ml/7fl oz/scant 1 cup skimmed (lowfat) milk
200ml/7fl oz/scant 1 cup water
4 tsp low-fat plain yogurt, to serve

**For the spiced fruit compôte**
200ml/7fl oz/scant 1 cup water
1 tsp runny honey
1 cinnamon stick
1 raspberry fruit tea bag
100g/3½oz mixed dried fruit, such as apricots, apples, peaches and pears

Serves 2
Prep: 5 minutes
Cook: 20 minutes

Make the fruit compôte: put the water, honey and cinnamon stick in a saucepan and bring to the boil. Reduce the heat, add the tea bag and simmer gently for 5 minutes.

Stir in the dried fruit and simmer for a further 10–15 minutes until softened. Remove and discard the tea bag.

Put the oats, salt, milk and water into a non-stick saucepan and bring to the bowl, stirring with a wooden spoon. Reduce the heat to a simmer and cook until the porridge is thick and really smooth. Stir occasionally to prevent it sticking and to break down any lumps.

Divide the porridge between two serving bowls and top with the warm fruit compôte and a swirl of yogurt.

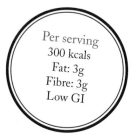

Per serving
300 kcals
Fat: 3g
Fibre: 3g
Low GI

# TUNA EGGS BENEDICT

Traditional eggs Benedict are served with grilled bacon or cooked ham, but tuna makes a healthier alternative. Keep a jar of extra-light mayonnaise in the refrigerator – it's so useful for sandwiches or adding a spoonful to fromage frais and yogurt dips. A tablespoon of extra-light mayo can be as low as 9 calories, compared with anything between 45 and a massive 240 for full-fat mayonnaise! You know it makes sense.

1 x 200g/7oz can tuna in spring water, drained
1 tbsp extra-light mayonnaise
2 tsp white wine vinegar
2 medium free-range eggs
1 wholemeal muffin, sliced in half
2 tbsp ready-made hollandaise sauce
few fresh chives, chopped
freshly ground black pepper

Serves 2
Prep: 10 minutes
Cook: 4–5 minutes

Use a fork to mash the tuna lightly with the mayonnaise in a bowl.

Half-fill a medium saucepan with water and place over a low heat until it is just simmering. Add the vinegar and then carefully break the eggs into the hot water. Leave them to poach in the gently simmering water for about 4 minutes until the whites are set but the yolks are still runny.

Meanwhile, toast the muffin lightly and divide the mashed tuna mixture equally between the two halves.

Heat the hollandaise sauce in a small saucepan over a very low heat until it is warm, then stir in the chopped chives.

Remove the eggs from the pan with a slotted spoon and drain well, then pat dry with kitchen paper. Place a poached egg on top of each tuna-topped muffin and drizzle the warm hollandaise sauce over the top. Season with a little black pepper and serve immediately.

Per serving
300 kcals
Fat: 16g
Fibre: 2g
Medium GI

SLIM FACT...
TUNA CANNED IN SPRING WATER HAS ONLY 108 CALORIES AND 0.6G FAT PER 100G/3½OZ, COMPARED WITH 188 CALORIES AND 9G FAT FOR TUNA CANNED IN OIL.

# SPANISH BAKED EGGS WITH CHORIZO

**This dish makes a spicy breakfast (without the salad) at the weekend or an easy supper. It's a variation on the Mexican classic** *huevos rancheros* **in which the eggs are cooked with tomatoes, peppers and chillies. Spicy chorizo sausage is extremely high in fat; however, it has a strong flavour, so you don't need much. In Spain it is cooked in a dry frying pan over a low to medium heat until all the fat runs out, and then it is added to salads.**

1 green (bell) pepper
1 yellow (bell) pepper
50g/1¾oz chorizo, diced
1 onion, chopped
1 garlic clove, crushed
1 x 200g/7oz can chopped tomatoes
1 tsp paprika
150ml/¼ pint/⅔ cup chicken or vegetable stock
salt and freshly ground black pepper
2 free-range eggs
few fresh parsley sprigs, chopped
2 handfuls of crisp green salad leaves
2 tsp oil-free vinaigrette dressing

Serves 2
Prep: 15 minutes
Cook: 45–50 minutes

Preheat the oven to 180°C/350°F/Gas mark 4.

Roast the peppers in the oven for 15–20 minutes until they soften and their skin blisters. Remove from the oven and leave to cool. When they are cool enough to handle, peel, core and deseed them, then cut the flesh into fine strips.

Meanwhile, cook the chorizo in a non-stick saucepan over a low heat, until the fat is released. Drain off the fat and then add the onion and garlic to the pan and cook over a medium heat until softened and golden.

Reduce the heat, add the tomatoes, pepper strips, paprika and stock and cook gently until the mixture reduces and thickens. Season to taste with salt and pepper. Divide the mixture between two ovenproof dishes. Make a small hollow in each one and crack a whole egg into the centre. Bake in the oven for about 10 minutes, or until the egg is cooked and set.

Serve immediately sprinkled with chopped parsley, and with crisp green salad leaves lightly dressed in oil-free vinaigrette.

Per serving
300 kcals
Fat: 14g
Fibre: 5g
Medium GI

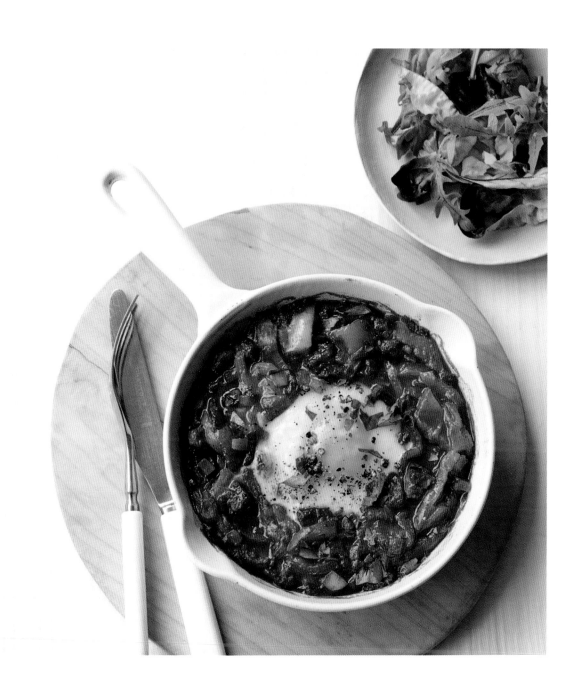

# SPICY BLACK BEAN SOUP

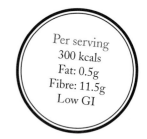

Per serving
300 kcals
Fat: 0.5g
Fibre: 11.5g
Low GI

**Soups made with black beans and vegetables, laced with chilli and spices, are made throughout the Caribbean and Mexico. They are filling, delicious and high in fibre, making them ideal for slimming and weight maintenance programmes. It's best to make your own salsa, as below, but you can cheat and use reduced-fat salsa, although it won't taste as good.**

spray oil
1 onion, chopped
2 garlic cloves, crushed
1 fresh red chilli, deseeded and finely diced
pinch of smoked sweet paprika
1 x 400g/14oz can black beans, drained and rinsed
1 x 400g/14oz can chopped tomatoes
400ml/14fl oz/1¾ cups vegetable stock
freshly ground black pepper
2 tbsp virtually fat-free fromage frais

**For the hot salsa garnish**
1 large tomato, diced
¼ red onion, finely chopped
1 red chilli, deseeded and finely diced
juice of 1 lime
few fresh coriander (cilantro) sprigs, chopped

Serves 2
Prep: 15 minutes
Cook: 30–35 minutes

Lightly spray a saucepan with oil and place over a low heat. Add the onion and garlic and cook gently for 10 minutes, or until softened and golden.

Add the chilli, paprika and most of the drained black beans, reserving a few for the salsa garnish. Cook for 1 minute, then stir in the chopped tomatoes and the stock. Bring to the boil, then reduce the heat and simmer gently for 15–20 minutes. Season to taste with pepper.

Meanwhile, mix all the salsa ingredients together with the reserved black beans.

Pour the soup into a blender or food processor and blitz until thick and smooth. Return to the pan and heat through gently.

Ladle the hot soup into two shallow bowls and swirl in the fromage frais. Top with the hot salsa garnish and serve.

COOK'S TIP...
THIS SOUP CAN BE MADE IN LARGER QUANTITIES – JUST DOUBLE OR TREBLE THE INGREDIENTS – AND THEN COOLED BEFORE FREEZING IN INDIVIDUAL PORTIONS. LABEL THEM WITH THE NAME AND CALORIE COUNT.

# FRENCH ONION SOUP

**A classic soup that is very low in fat and calories if it's made without the usual quantities of oil, butter and sugar. Reduced-fat Cheddar cheese has less than half the fat (16.7g compared to 33.2g per 100g/3½oz) of regular full-fat Cheddar, and 270 calories versus 404. Even if you're just sprinkling a tablespoon of grated cheese over a gratin or soup, it all adds up and makes a difference.**

spray oil
2 large onions, thinly sliced
2 bay leaves
2 tsp plain (all-purpose) flour
500ml/18fl oz/generous 2 cups hot vegetable stock
75ml/2½fl oz/5 tbsp dry white wine
sea salt and freshly ground black pepper

For the cheese croûtes:
2 x 30g/1oz slices baguette
1 tsp Dijon mustard
2 tbsp grated reduced-fat Cheddar cheese

Serves 2
Prep: 10 minutes
Cook: 55 minutes

Lightly spray a large heavy-based saucepan with oil and place over a medium heat. When it's hot, add the onions and bay leaves and cook very gently for 15–20 minutes, stirring occasionally to prevent them sticking, until the onions are really tender and starting to caramelize.

Stir in the flour and cook for 1 minute, then add the hot stock and wine. Increase the heat and bring to the boil. Season to taste with salt and pepper, then reduce the heat to a bare simmer and cook gently for 30 minutes.

Preheat the grill (broiler). Just before serving the soup, toast the slices of bread on one side only. Spread the untoasted sides with Dijon mustard and then sprinkle with grated cheese.

Divide the hot soup between two heatproof shallow bowls and float the croûtes, cheese-side up, in the soup. Pop the bowls under the hot grill for a couple of minutes or so until the cheese melts appetizingly. Serve immediately.

Per serving
300 kcals
Fat: 4g
Fibre: 3.5g
Medium GI

# THAI PRAWN AND VEGETABLE SOUP

**Substantial soups such as this one make a complete meal in a bowl, and they're surprisingly simple to prepare and quick to cook. This soup is very refreshing and packed with interesting flavours, which all complement each other. You can vary the vegetables, using mangetout (snow peas) instead of sugar snap peas, spring greens (collard greens) instead of pak choi and Thai basil instead of coriander.**

spray oil
1 garlic clove, crushed
1 small red chilli, deseeded and sliced
1 tsp grated fresh root ginger
1 lemongrass stalk, peeled and diced
4 spring onions (scallions), sliced
1 carrot, cut into matchsticks
1 red (bell) pepper, cut into thin strips
1 kaffir lime leaf (optional)
100ml/3½fl oz/scant ½ cup reduced-fat coconut milk
300ml/½ pint/1¼ cups vegetable stock
200g/7oz peeled raw tiger prawns (jumbo shrimp)
1 head pak choi (bok choy), sliced
85g/3oz sugar snap peas, sliced
100g/3½oz/scant 1 cup frozen peas
125g/4½oz dried rice noodles
1 tsp nam pla (Thai fish sauce)
juice of ½ lime
few fresh coriander (cilantro) sprigs, roughly chopped

Serves 2
Prep: 15 minutes
Cook: 15 minutes

Lightly spray a pan with oil and place over a high heat. When it's really hot, add the garlic, chilli, ginger, lemongrass and two spring onions and stir-fry for 30 seconds.

Add the carrot and red pepper and stir-fry for 30 seconds, then stir in the lime leaf (if using), coconut milk and stock. Reduce the heat and simmer gently for 5 minutes.

Add the prawns, pak choi, sugar snaps and peas and simmer gently for 5 minutes, or until the prawns turn pink and the vegetables are tender.

Meanwhile, cook the rice noodles according to the packet instructions, then drain.

Stir the cooked rice noodles, nam pla and lime juice into the soup. Heat through gently and then ladle the soup into deep bowls. Sprinkle with chopped coriander and the remaining spring onions and serve immediately.

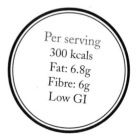

Per serving
300 kcals
Fat: 6.8g
Fibre: 6g
Low GI

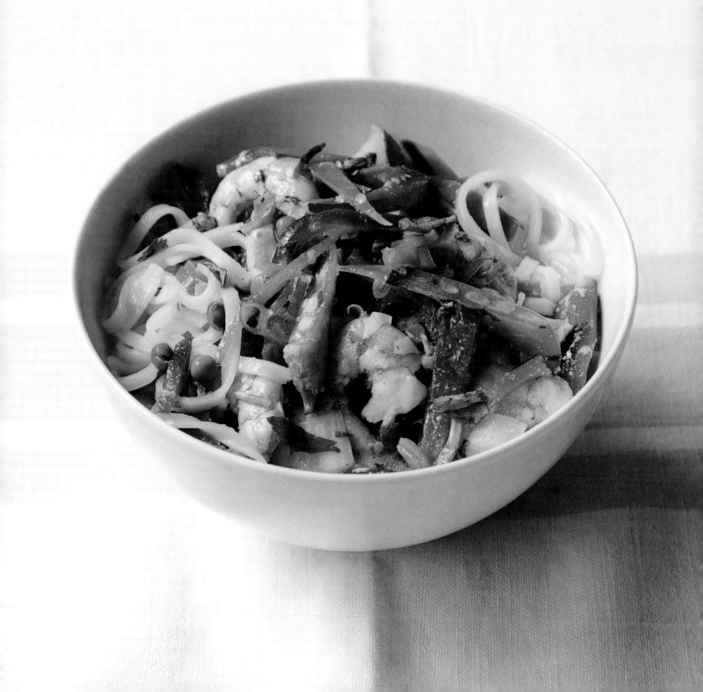

# NOODLES WITH SPICED CRAB AND LEMON

**You can buy ready-cooked crabs from good fishmongers and most supermarkets' fresh fish counters. Crab is strongly flavoured and a little goes a long way in a dish like this. If you love lemons, you can add the grated zest, too. For a more Asian touch, try chopped fresh coriander (cilantro) leaves instead of parsley.**

100g/3½oz dried tagliatelle or fettuccine
spray olive oil
3 garlic cloves, crushed
1 small red chilli, finely chopped
50ml/2fl oz/scant ¼ cup dry white wine
juice of 1 lemon
125g/4½oz cooked crabmeat
1 small bunch of fresh parsley, chopped
salt and freshly ground black pepper
watercress or rocket (arugula) leaves, to serve

Serves 2
Prep: 5 minutes
Cook: 10 minutes

Cook the pasta in a large saucepan of boiling salted water according to the packet instructions until it is just tender but still retains some bite (al dente). Drain well.

While the pasta is cooking, lightly spray a large frying pan with oil and quickly cook the garlic and chilli over a medium heat for 1–2 minutes. Add the wine and lemon juice and cook for a few minutes until the wine reduces and releases its flavour and aroma.

Stir in the crabmeat and chopped parsley and season to taste with salt and pepper. Heat through gently.

Toss the cooked pasta in the crab mixture until it's well coated. Serve immediately with watercress or rocket leaves.

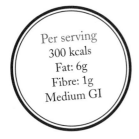

Per serving
300 kcals
Fat: 6g
Fibre: 1g
Medium GI

# STIR-FRIED CHILLI BEEF

**It's important that you use egg noodles in this delicious spicy stir-fry; they have 62 calories per 100g/3½oz cooked weight compared to 109 calories for cooked rice noodles. You can vary the vegetables, substituting yellow or green pepper and sugar snaps or mangetout for the red pepper and carrot.**

250g/9oz lean sirloin (porterhouse) steak, all visible fat removed

pinch of ground Szechuan peppercorns

spray oil

1 fresh red chilli, finely sliced

2 garlic cloves, crushed

1 tsp grated fresh root ginger

1 carrot, cut into matchsticks

1 large celery stick, cut into matchsticks

1 red (bell) pepper, deseeded and thinly sliced

pinch of five-spice powder

1 tbsp soy sauce

1 tsp hoisin sauce

250g/9oz fresh Chinese egg noodles, boiled and drained

**To garnish**

2 spring onions (scallions), shredded

fresh coriander (cilantro) leaves

Serves 2

Prep: 10 minutes

Cook: 5–10 minutes

Slice the steak into thin strips and season them generously with the Szechuan pepper.

Lightly spray a wok or deep frying pan with oil and set over a medium heat. When it's hot, add the steak strips and stir-fry for 1 minute until the steak is seared all over.

Add the chilli, garlic, ginger, carrot, celery, red pepper and five-spice powder and stir-fry briskly for 2 minutes. Stir in the soy and hoisin sauces and cook for a further 2 minutes. Gently stir in the cooked egg noodles and warm through quickly.

Divide between two shallow serving bowls and serve immediately sprinkled with shredded spring onion and coriander.

OR TRY THIS...
YOU CAN STIR-FRY PORK IN THE SAME WAY. USE 200G/7OZ VERY LEAN PORK TENDERLOIN (FILLET) AND REMOVE ANY VISIBLE FAT BEFORE COOKING.

Per serving
300 kcals
Fat: 8.5g
Fibre: 3.5g
Medium GI

# SPRING VEGETABLE LASAGNE STACKS

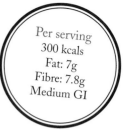

Per serving
300 kcals
Fat: 7g
Fibre: 7.8g
Medium GI

**In this recipe, the lasagne stacks are assembled on the serving plates just before eating. Cook dry lasagne sheets in a very large saucepan with plenty of boiling water to prevent them sticking together. Fresh lasagne is quicker to cook and the sheets won't stick.**

4 x 20g/¾oz sheets fresh or dried lasagne

250g/9oz baby spinach leaves

200g/7oz/scant 1 cup extra-light soft cheese

a pinch of grated nutmeg

grated zest of 1 lemon

15g/½oz sunblush tomatoes, drained and chopped

salt and freshly ground black pepper

200g/7oz baby courgettes (zucchini), sliced lengthways

200g/7oz asparagus, trimmed

2 x 100g/3½oz bunches of cherry tomatoes on the vine

good balsamic vinegar, for drizzling

few fresh chives, to garnish

Serves 2
Prep: 15 minutes
Cook: 10 minutes

Cook the lasagne sheets in a large saucepan of boiling salted water for 8–10 minutes, or according to the packet instructions, until tender. Remove the sheets carefully with a slotted spoon so as not to break them, and drain well.

Meanwhile, put the spinach in a saucepan with a teaspoonful of water and cook over a medium heat for 2 minutes, stirring and shaking the pan, until it wilts and turns bright green. Drain well, pressing it down with a saucer in a colander to extract all the moisture. Mix with the soft cheese, nutmeg, lemon zest, sunblush tomatoes and pepper, then season with salt to taste, if needed.

Preheat the grill (broiler). Steam the courgettes for a few minutes until just tender, then remove from the heat. Boil or steam the asparagus for about 6 minutes until just tender. Drain.

Grill the cherry tomatoes for a few minutes until softened and slightly charred.

Cut each pasta sheet in half. Place one piece on each serving plate and spread with a little of the spinach mixture and some courgette and asparagus. Cover with another sheet of lasagne and continue layering up in this way, so you end up with four sheets in each stack.

Drizzle a little balsamic vinegar over the top of each stack and garnish with chives. Serve immediately with the grilled cherry tomatoes.

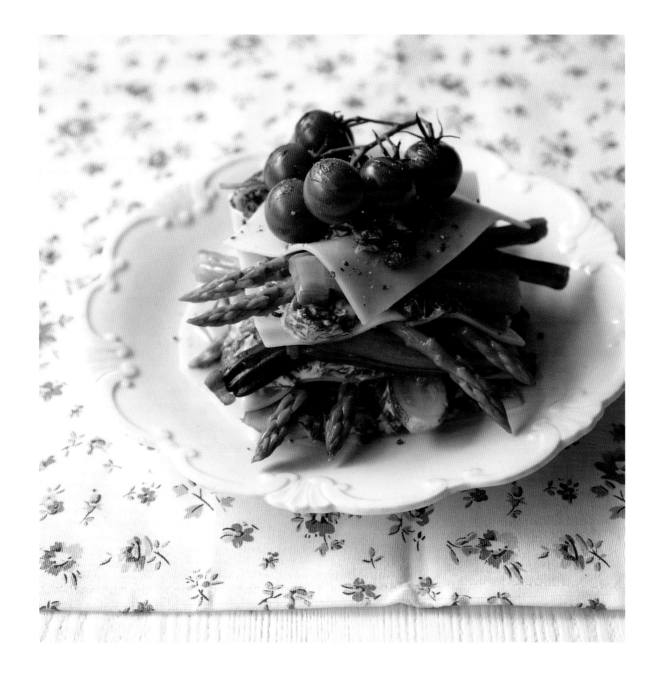

# LEMONY PRIMAVERA RISOTTO

**Risotto is the ultimate comfort food, but it can be high in fat and calories if it is made in the traditional way with butter. This one, however, is full of fresh green vegetables and flavoured with lemon and herbs; it's the perfect supper for a spring or summer evening.**

spray olive oil
1 onion, finely chopped
2 garlic cloves, crushed
100g/3½oz baby leeks, trimmed
pinch of chilli powder
100g/3½oz/scant ½ cup arborio or
carnaroli risotto rice
2 tbsp dry white wine or vermouth,
such as Noilly Prat
400ml/14fl oz/1¾ cups hot
vegetable stock
few saffron strands (optional)
50g/1¾oz/scant ½ cup frozen peas
50g/1¾oz baby asparagus
2 small courgettes (zucchini), sliced
grated zest and juice of 1 lemon
salt and freshly ground black pepper
small bunch of fresh flat-leaf
parsley, chopped
1 tbsp grated Parmesan cheese

Serves 2
Prep: 10 minutes
Cook: 30 minutes

Lightly spray a large deep frying pan with oil and place over a low heat. Add the onion and garlic and cook gently, stirring occasionally, for 10 minutes until tender and translucent, but not browned.

Add the baby leeks and cook for 2 minutes. Stir in the chilli powder and risotto rice. Cook for 1 minute and then add the wine or vermouth. It will hiss and bubble briefly. Then cook for 3–4 minutes until reduced.

Stir in the saffron and start adding the hot stock, a ladleful at a time. Cook very gently, stirring in more stock a little at a time, waiting for the rice to absorb it before adding more, for about 15 minutes, until the rice is just tender but still slightly resistant to the bite. Stir frequently to prevent the rice sticking to the pan.

Add the peas, asparagus and courgettes and cook for 5 minutes, or until tender. Stir in the lemon zest and juice and remove from the heat. Season to taste with salt and pepper, then stir in the parsley.

Leave the risotto to stand for 5 minutes, then sprinkle with the grated Parmesan and serve immediately.

Per serving
300 kcals
Fat: 3g
Fibre: 6.5g
Medium GI

# GRILLED SPICED BEEF WITH TABBOULEH

Per serving
300 kcals
Fat: 8g
Fibre: 4.5g
Medium GI

**Nutty-textured bulgur wheat is a good dietary source of protein and minerals. It's so easy to prepare and you can mix it with chopped fresh herbs, tomatoes, olives, onions and lemon or lime juice to make a delicious Middle Eastern salad. It's particularly good served with grilled meat, chicken or falafel.**

225g/8oz beef fillet (tenderloin), all visible fat removed
2 tbsp soy sauce
pinch of ground star anise
1 garlic clove, crushed
1 tsp finely chopped fresh root ginger
grated zest of 1 lemon
freshly ground black pepper
spray olive oil
crisp lettuce leaves, to serve

**For the tabbouleh**
75g/2¾oz/½ cup bulgur wheat
¼ cucumber, diced
2 ripe tomatoes, diced
2 spring onions (scallions), finely sliced
few fresh parsley sprigs, chopped
1 handful of fresh mint, chopped
juice of 1 lemon
2 tbsp oil-free vinaigrette dressing

Serves 2
Prep: 20 minutes
Marinate: 12 hours
Soak: 15–20 minutes
Cook: 8–12 minutes

Put the beef in a shallow dish. Stir the soy sauce, star anise, garlic, ginger and lemon zest together in a bowl, then sprinkle over the beef. Season with pepper, then cover and leave to marinate in the refrigerator for at least 12 hours.

Make the tabbouleh: put the bulgur wheat in a heatproof bowl and pour enough boiling water over to cover it. Leave to soak for 15–20 minutes until it swells up and absorbs the liquid. Squeeze out any excess moisture. Stir in the prepared vegetables, herbs, lemon juice and dressing.

Lightly spray a ridged griddle pan with oil. Lift the beef out of the marinade and cook over a high heat for about 4–6 minutes on each side, depending on how well cooked you like your beef. Ideally, it should be seared on the outside and pink and juicy inside. Leave to rest for 5 minutes.

Carve the beef into thin slices and serve immediately with the tabbouleh and some crisp lettuce.

OR TRY THIS...
USE DIFFERENT FLAVOURINGS FOR THE TABBOULEH, SUCH AS CHOPPED CORIANDER (CILANTRO), FINELY DICED RED ONION, LIME JUICE, OR CHILLI. IF ADDING OLIVES, PROCEED WITH CAUTION – A SINGLE 3G OLIVE CAN VARY BETWEEN 4 AND 9 CALORIES. BLACK OLIVES ARE HIGHER IN CALORIES AND FAT THAN GREEN ONES.

# WARM ROASTED SQUASH AND LENTIL SALAD

**You will need Puy lentils or ordinary green or brown ones for this salad because they retain their shape after cooking. The red or yellow split lentils will turn to mush when cooked and are not suitable. If you don't like the taste of goat's cheese, you can substitute the same weight of diced reduced-fat mozzarella.**

200g/7oz butternut squash, peeled, deseeded and cubed
1 red onion, cut into thin wedges
1 small red (bell) pepper, deseeded and diced
spray olive oil
100g/3½oz/½ cup Puy lentils
salt and freshly ground black pepper
few fresh parsley sprigs, chopped
drizzle of balsamic vinegar
50g/1¾oz wild rocket (arugula)
60g/2¼oz goat's cheese, crumbled

Serves 2
Prep: 10 minutes
Cook: 35 minutes

Preheat the oven to 200°C/400°F/Gas mark 6.

Spread the butternut squash cubes on a non-stick baking sheet with the red onion and red pepper. Spray lightly with oil and roast in the oven for 30–35 minutes, turning occasionally, until tender.

Meanwhile, put the lentils in a saucepan and cover them with cold water. Bring to the boil, then reduce the heat and simmer gently for 15–20 minutes until they are cooked but not mushy – they should still retain a little 'bite'. Drain well.

Put the warm roasted vegetables and lentils in a large bowl and season to taste with salt and pepper. Stir in the parsley and drizzle with balsamic vinegar. Leave for 5 minutes to allow the flavours to develop.

Stir the rocket and goat's cheese into the salad and serve immediately.

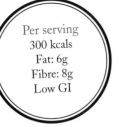

Per serving
300 kcals
Fat: 6g
Fibre: 8g
Low GI

OR TRY THIS…
THIS SALAD LOOKS AND TASTES GREAT SERVED WITH BABY PLUM TOMATOES. AN AVERAGE 50G/1¾OZ SERVING WILL ADD 9 CALORIES.

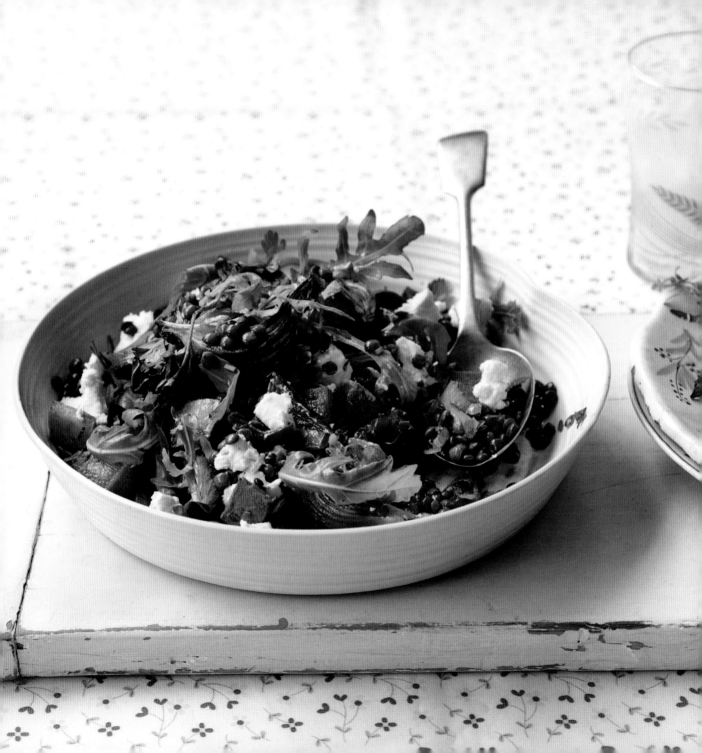

# SPANISH ROASTED PEPPER AND SPINACH TORTILLA

The beauty of this dish is that it can be served for brunch, lunch or dinner and eaten warm or cold. Wrap it in foil and take it to work with you for a delicious packed lunch. In Spain, tortilla is often cut into small squares and served cold with drinks as tapas. Eggs are high in protein and low in calories, but they contain a lot of fat – an average of 6g per medium egg, so you may wish to moderate your intake if you're on a low-fat regime.

2 yellow (bell) peppers
spray olive oil
1 red onion, thinly sliced
250g/9oz waxy potatoes, scrubbed or peeled and diced
150g/5½oz baby spinach leaves
3 free-range eggs, beaten
salt and freshly ground black pepper

Serves 2
Prep: 15 minutes
Cook: 30 minutes

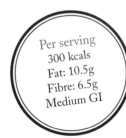

Per serving
300 kcals
Fat: 10.5g
Fibre: 6.5g
Medium GI

Preheat the grill (broiler). Put the yellow peppers on a grill pan and cook under the hot grill, turning them occasionally, until the skins start to blister and char. Remove from the heat and leave to cool.

Peel the peppers and remove and discard the stalks, seeds and ribs. Cut the flesh into thin strips.

Lightly spray a non-stick, ovenproof frying pan with oil and place over a medium heat. When it's hot, add the onion and potatoes and cook, stirring frequently, for about 10–15 minutes until the potatoes are tender and golden brown, and the onion starts to caramelize.

Stir in the pepper strips and spinach and cook for 2–3 minutes until the spinach turns bright green and wilts.

Pour in the beaten eggs, and salt and pepper, tilting the pan to cover the bottom and sides evenly. Reduce the heat to a bare simmer and cook gently for about 5 minutes, or until the tortilla is set and golden underneath.

Meanwhile, preheat the grill. Pop the tortilla pan under the hot grill until the top of the tortilla is set and golden brown. Slide it out of the pan and cut in half to serve.

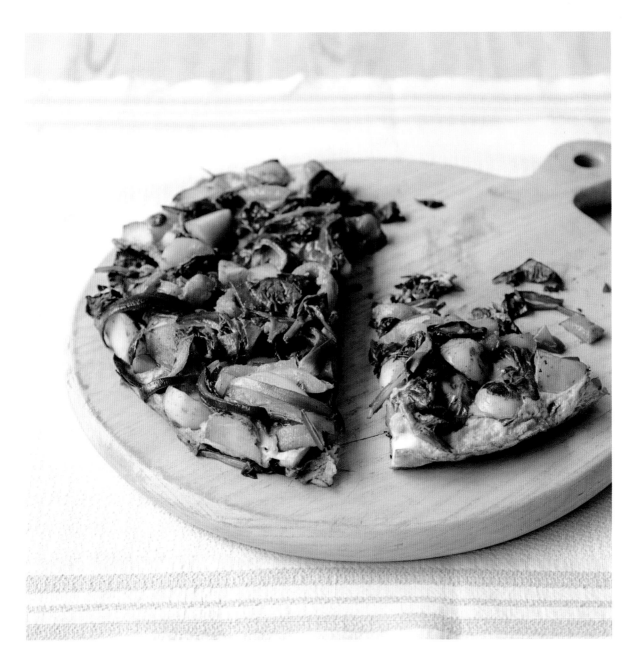

# PRAWN
## CAESAR SALAD

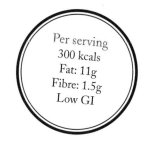

Per serving
300 kcals
Fat: 11g
Fibre: 1.5g
Low GI

Caesar salad – the ultimate salad for garlic lovers – is deceptively filling and makes a quick and easy supper on a warm summer's evening. You can use cooked prawns instead of the raw ones here, but they won't taste as good. If using ready-bought croûtons, check the labels carefully to buy the lowest-calorie version on sale – some are much higher in fat than others.

spray oil

2 garlic cloves, crushed

juice of ½ lemon

200g/7oz peeled raw tiger prawns (jumbo shrimp) (fresh or frozen and thawed)

2 tbsp finely chopped fresh parsley

1 head cos (romaine) lettuce, roughly shredded

2 tbsp salad croûtons

2 tbsp grated Parmesan cheese

**For the Caesar dressing**

2 tbsp oil-free vinaigrette dressing

grated zest and juice of 1 lemon

1 large garlic clove, crushed

few drops of Worcestershire sauce

1 raw small free-range egg yolk

salt and freshly ground black pepper

Serves 2

Prep: 15 minutes

Cook: 6–8 minutes

Lightly spray a frying pan with oil and place over a medium heat. When it's hot, add the garlic and stir-fry for 1 minute until softened but not browned.

Pour in the lemon juice and let it bubble away for a minute or so before adding the prawns. Cook briskly for 3–4 minutes, turning them halfway through, until they are pink on both sides. Sprinkle with parsley and remove the pan from the heat.

Make the Caesar dressing: mix the vinaigrette dressing, lemon zest and juice, garlic and Worcestershire sauce together in a bowl. Beat in the egg yolk and season to taste with salt and pepper.

Toss the lettuce and croûtons in the dressing and divide the salad between two serving plates. Arrange the hot prawns on top and pour over any pan juices. Sprinkle with the grated Parmesan cheese and serve immediately.

NOTE:
IF YOU ARE PREGNANT, ELDERLY OR UNWELL, YOU SHOULD OMIT THE RAW EGG YOLK FROM THE DRESSING.

# GREEK GRILLED HALLOUMI AND VEGETABLES

**Always opt for light halloumi cheese: it has 16g of fat per 100g compared to 24.7g for regular halloumi. Its firm texture and slightly salty taste makes it a great choice for salads. This grilled version of the classic Greek *horiatiki* salad with added chickpeas is surprisingly substantial and filling.**

spray olive oil

1 garlic clove, crushed

1 small aubergine (eggplant), cubed

1 small red (bell) pepper, deseeded and cut into chunks

2 vine tomatoes, halved

200g/7oz canned chickpeas, rinsed and drained

½ red onion, very thinly sliced

4 small black olives, pitted

100g/3½oz light halloumi cheese

1 tbsp oil-free vinaigrette dressing

grated zest and juice of 1 lemon

few fresh mint or parsley sprigs, chopped

freshly ground black pepper

Serves 2

Prep: 10 minutes

Cook: 17 minutes

Lightly spray a ridged griddle pan with oil. Place over a medium heat, add the garlic, aubergine and red pepper and cook for 8–10 minutes, turning them occasionally, until softened.

Add the tomatoes and cook for 4–5 minutes or until everything is tender but still retains a little bite. Don't worry if the vegetables are slightly charred.

Mix the chickpeas with the red onion and olives. Add the grilled vegetables and divide between two serving plates.

Cut the halloumi into four slices and cook in the hot pan for 2 minutes, or until golden brown on both sides.

Mix the vinaigrette with the lemon zest and juice and chopped herbs and drizzle over the salad. Place the hot halloumi slices on top. Grind over a little pepper and serve immediately.

OR TRY THIS...
INSTEAD OF HALLOUMI, TRY SOME SALTY FETA CHEESE. SUBSTITUTE 90G/3¼OZ FETA, CUT INTO CUBES. THE CALORIES WILL STAY THE SAME, BUT THE FAT CONTENT WILL INCREASE BY 1G PER SERVING.

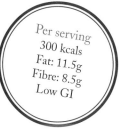

Per serving
300 kcals
Fat: 11.5g
Fibre: 8.5g
Low GI

# ITALIAN LENTIL AND MOZZARELLA SALAD

**Lentils are high in fibre as well as protein and they really do fill you up when you're on a diet and trying to eat more healthily. Instead of serving them lukewarm or cold with mozzarella, as suggested below, you can also eat the lentils hot, sprinkled with 3 tablespoons grated Parmesan cheese.**

100g/3½oz/½ cup Puy or green lentils
spray oil
1 small onion, chopped
1 large carrot, finely diced
2 celery sticks, diced
2 garlic cloves, crushed
100g/3½oz baby plum tomatoes, halved
juice of 1 lemon
few fresh basil sprigs, finely torn, plus extra leaves to garnish
salt and freshly ground black pepper
100g/3½oz fine green beans, trimmed
1 tbsp oil-free vinaigrette dressing
1 tbsp balsamic vinegar, plus extra for drizzling
85g/3oz reduced-fat mozzarella, thinly sliced or torn into pieces

Serves 2
Prep: 10 minutes
Cook: 30 minutes

Put the lentils in a saucepan and cover them with cold water. Bring to the boil, then reduce the heat and simmer gently for 20–25 minutes until they are tender but still have a little bite. Drain and refresh under cold running water.

Meanwhile, spray a large frying pan lightly with oil and place over a low heat. Add the onion, carrot, celery and garlic and sweat them gently until they are soft and translucent.

Add the tomatoes and lentils and cook for 5 minutes, stirring occasionally. If the lentils start to stick, add a little water. Stir in the lemon juice and torn basil leaves and season to taste with salt and pepper. Remove from the heat and leave to cool slightly.

Cook the green beans in a saucepan of boiling water for 3–4 minutes. Drain and refresh under cold running water.

Stir the vinaigrette dressing and balsamic vinegar into the lentil mixture and divide between two serving plates – it should be lukewarm or you can leave it and serve at room temperature. Top with the mozzarella and green beans. Drizzle with some more balsamic vinegar, if wished, and garnish with a few basil leaves.

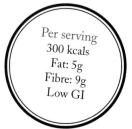

Per serving
300 kcals
Fat: 5g
Fibre: 9g
Low GI

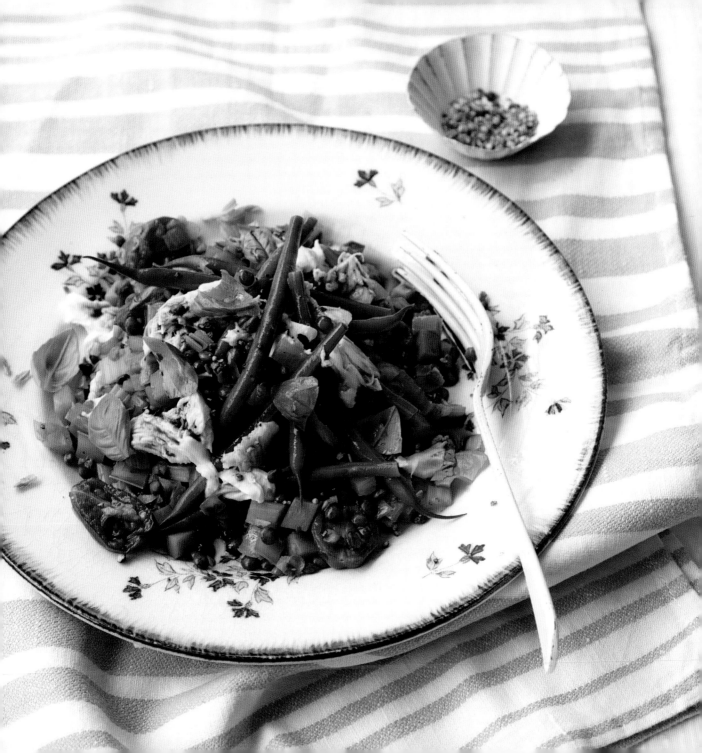

# BULGUR WHEAT SALAD WITH ROASTED VEGETABLES

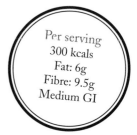

Per serving
300 kcals
Fat: 6g
Fibre: 9.5g
Medium GI

A colourful salad of nutty-tasting bulgur wheat with roasted vegetables and salty feta. It's served with fiery red Moroccan harissa paste; you need only a dab as it is so hot! If you can find it, buy reduced-fat feta, which averages out at about 25 calories and 4g fat per 30g/1oz. The same quantity of regular feta contains 75 calories and 6g fat. So you could triple the amount used in the recipe below and still have a 300-calorie supper.

100g/3½oz/¾ cup bulgur wheat
1 small fennel bulb, trimmed and cut into large pieces
1 yellow courgette (zucchini), cut into chunks
1 small red onion, cut into chunks
1 small red (bell) pepper, cut into chunks
1 small green (bell) pepper, cut into chunks
2 unpeeled garlic cloves
spray olive oil
salt and freshly ground black pepper
few drops of balsamic vinegar
few fresh flat-leaf parsley sprigs, chopped
few fresh mint sprigs, chopped
few fresh basil leaves, chopped
50g/1¾oz feta cheese, cubed
juice of 1 lemon
dash of harissa paste, to serve

Serves 2
Prep: 20 minutes
Soak: 20 minutes
Cook: 30–35 minutes

Preheat the oven to 200°C/400°F/ Gas mark 6.

Put the bulgur wheat in a bowl and cover with cold water. Leave to soak for 20 minutes.

Put all the vegetables, including the garlic, in a single layer in a large roasting pan. Spray lightly with oil and season with salt and pepper. Roast in the oven for 30–35 minutes, turning them once or twice, until they are tender and starting to char round the edges.

Remove from the oven and sprinkle the hot vegetables with a few drops of balsamic vinegar. Leave to cool.

Meanwhile, drain the bulgur wheat and put it in a saucepan. Cover with cold water and bring to the boil. Reduce the heat and simmer gently for 15 minutes. Drain well and put the bulgur wheat in a serving bowl. Gently mix in the roasted vegetables, herbs and feta. Sprinkle with lemon juice and serve warm with a little harissa paste.

# BAJA GRIDDLED CHICKEN SALAD

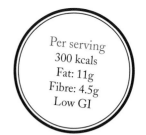

This main course salad resonates with the spicy flavours and colourful vegetables of the Baja peninsula in southern California. Use a baby avocado (200 calories) for the guacamole – a large avocado can pack up to 700 calories.

spray olive oil
1 red (bell) pepper, cut into chunks
1 yellow (bell) pepper, cut into chunks
2 x 100g/3½oz skinless, boneless chicken breasts
1 head crisp cos (romaine) lettuce
few fresh coriander (cilantro) sprigs
4 pickled chillies
2 tbsp oil-free vinaigrette dressing
1 tsp balsamic vinegar
1 tsp sweet chilli sauce
pinch of paprika, for dusting

**For the guacamole**
1 baby avocado, peeled and stoned
1 large ripe tomato, diced
¼ red onion, finely diced
1 small red or green chilli, deseeded and diced
juice of 1 lime
50g/1¾oz/scant ¼ cup virtually fat-free fromage frais
handful of fresh coriander (cilantro) leaves, chopped

Serves 2
Prep: 15 minutes
Cook: 15–20 minutes

Lightly spray a ridged griddle pan and place over a medium heat. When it's hot, add the peppers and chicken and cook for 15–20 minutes, turning occasionally, until the peppers are tender and charred and the chicken is golden brown and cooked right through. To test, pierce the thickest part of the flesh with a thin skewer; the juices should run golden, not pink.

While they are cooking, mash the avocado and mix all the ingredients for the guacamole together in a bowl.

Tear the lettuce leaves in half, then mix them in a bowl with the coriander, pickled chillies and grilled peppers. Divide the salad between two serving plates.

Slice the cooked chicken breasts and arrange on top of the salad. Combine the vinaigrette dressing, balsamic vinegar and chilli sauce together and drizzle over the chicken and salad.

Serve the salad immediately, dusted with paprika, with the guacamole.

OR TRY THIS...
AS WELL AS THE GUACAMOLE, YOU CAN SERVE THIS SALAD WITH LOW-FAT TOMATO SALSA (SEE PAGE 22) (16 CALORIES PER 50G/1¾OZ) AND SOME CREAMY VIRTUALLY FAT-FREE FROMAGE FRAIS OR 0% FAT GREEK YOGURT (APPROXIMATELY 7 CALORIES PER TABLESPOON).

# CHICKEN, MOZZARELLA AND PEPPER QUESADILLAS

**Mexican quesadillas are tortillas that are stuffed with a savoury filling and folded over to enclose it. They are usually filled with cheese or a mixture of cheese and vegetables, then served with tomato salsa and sometimes guacamole or soured cream. Our low-fat version has half the calories of most quesadillas.**

spray olive oil
150g/5½oz chicken breast fillets, skinned
1 red (bell) pepper, deseeded and cut into slices
1 green (bell) pepper, deseeded and cut into slices
2 tbsp low-fat tomato salsa (see page 22)
2 x 30g/1oz soft wholewheat tortillas
60g/2¼oz reduced-fat mozzarella cheese, thinly sliced

**To serve**
mixed salad leaves
few drops of balsamic vinegar

Serves 2
Prep: 10 minutes
Cook: 12 minutes

Spray a ridged griddle pan lightly with oil and place over a medium heat. When it's hot, add the chicken and peppers and cook for 5–6 minutes, turning them frequently, until the chicken is cooked through and golden brown, and the peppers have softened.

Cut the cooked chicken into chunks. Spread the salsa over the tortillas and top with the chicken, peppers and mozzarella. Fold each tortilla over to enclose the filling.

Put the griddle pan back on the heat and carefully place the filled tortillas in the hot pan. Heat through for 2–3 minutes on each side. Alternatively, you can pop them into the microwave for long enough to warm them through and melt the cheese.

Serve the quesadillas immediately with salad leaves drizzled with balsamic vinegar.

OR TRY THIS...
IF YOU WANT TO SERVE TRADITIONAL MEXICAN ACCOMPANIMENTS, CHOOSE REDUCED-FAT GUACAMOLE (22 CALORIES AND 2G FAT PER TABLESPOON) AND VIRTUALLY FAT-FREE FROMAGE FRAIS OR 0% FAT GREEK YOGURT (7 CALORIES PER TABLESPOON).

Per serving
300 kcals
Fat: 7.8g
Fibre: 5.5g
Medium GI

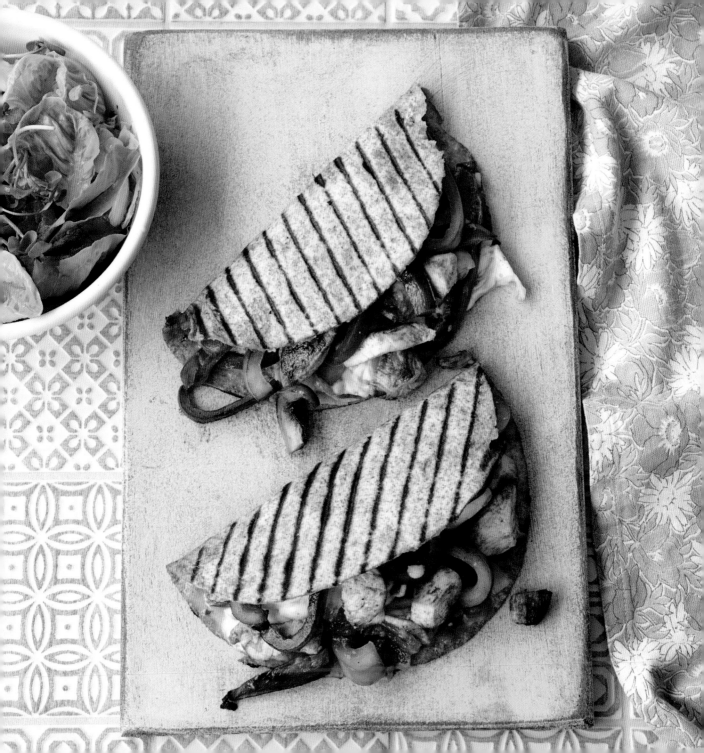

# SOUVLAKI PITTAS

**Souvlaki is a traditional Greek dish of skewered tender cuts of meat or chicken or meatballs. Here, minced lamb is subtly enhanced with herbs and spices and made into small meatballs for grilling – or cook on a hot barbecue for a really smoky flavour. These pittas can be eaten hot or cold and make a delicious packed lunch.**

200g/7oz extra lean minced (ground) lamb
1 tsp ground coriander
1 tbsp chopped fresh mint
1 tbsp chopped fresh oregano or pinch of dried
grated zest of 1 lemon
salt and freshly ground black pepper
2 x 45g/1½oz reduced-fat wholemeal pitta breads
50g/1¾oz salad leaves, such as cos (romaine) or rocket (arugula)

**For the tzatziki**
100g/3½oz/scant ½ cup low-fat plain yogurt
¼ cucumber, diced
1 garlic clove, crushed
juice of 1 small lemon
few fresh mint sprigs, chopped

Serves 2
Prep: 15 minutes
Cook: 10 minutes

Soak four small bamboo skewers in water for a few minutes to prevent them burning during cooking.

Preheat the grill (broiler). In a bowl, mix together the lamb, ground coriander, chopped herbs, lemon zest and seasoning. Divide the mixture into eight equal portions and mould each one into a ball with your hands.

Thread two lamb balls onto a skewer, then repeat the process with three more skewers.

Lay the kebabs on a foil-lined grill pan and cook under the hot grill for 8–10 minutes, turning them frequently, until they are cooked but still juicy.

While the lamb is cooking, mix all the ingredients for the tzatziki together in a bowl and season with pepper.

Warm and split the pitta breads and fill them with the meatballs and salad leaves topped with the tzatziki.

OR TRY THIS...
INSTEAD OF TZATZIKI, YOU COULD
TOP THE MEATBALLS WITH 30G/1OZ
REDUCED-FAT HUMMUS: THIS WILL
INCREASE THE FAT CONTENT BY
2G FAT PER SERVING.

Per serving
300 kcals
Fat: 7.5g
Fibre: 3g
Medium GI

# SCRAMBLED EGG AND PESTO TORTILLA WRAPS

**You can eat these tasty wraps for breakfast, brunch or lunch. Check the labels carefully when buying packs of tortillas – they vary hugely in their fat and calorie content. You are looking for 40–45g/1½oz tortilla wraps with a total of approximately 100 calories per wrap.**

3 medium free-range eggs
2 tbsp skimmed (lowfat) milk
salt and freshly ground black pepper
30g/1oz reduced-fat Cheddar cheese, grated
spray oil
2 x 45g/1½oz low-fat tortilla wraps
2 tsp low-fat green pesto
2 ripe tomatoes, diced

Serves 2
Prep: 10 minutes
Cook: 5 minutes

Whisk the eggs and milk together in a bowl. Season lightly with salt and pepper and stir in the grated cheese.

Lightly spray a small non-stick saucepan with oil and place over a very low heat. Add the beaten eggs and stir gently with a wooden spoon for a few minutes until they start to set and scramble. Do not overcook them or they will go watery.

Meanwhile, warm the tortilla wraps in a low oven or on a non-stick griddle pan. Spread the pesto over the warm tortillas and sprinkle with the diced tomatoes.

Spoon the scrambled egg on top and roll up or fold over to make a parcel, tucking in the ends. Eat immediately while the egg is still hot.

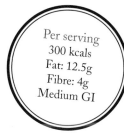

Per serving
300 kcals
Fat: 12.5g
Fibre: 4g
Medium GI

OR TRY THIS...
GIVE THESE TORTILLAS A TEX-MEX FLAVOUR BY OMITTING THE PESTO AND ADDING A LITTLE DICED RED CHILLI AND CHOPPED FRESH CORIANDER (CILANTRO) TO THE BEATEN EGGS BEFORE SCRAMBLING THEM. OMIT THE CHEESE FROM THE EGG MIXTURE AND SPRINKLE IT OVER THE TOMATOES AND EGGS AT THE END. THE CALORIES AND FAT COUNT WILL STAY THE SAME.

# QUICK PARMA HAM AND ROCKET PIZZAS

**You don't have to use regular pizza dough bases to make pizza – try using pitta breads instead, which are so simple and much lower in calories. Try pitta breads instead. They are simple to use and lower in calories. If you don't have any bottled peppers in your store cupboard, you can use a finely sliced fresh small yellow pepper instead.**

4 tbsp passata (strained tomatoes)
2 x 60g/2¼oz wholemeal pitta breads
50g/1¾oz bottled red and yellow pepper strips, drained
½ red onion, thinly sliced
100g/3½oz mushrooms, thinly sliced
50g/1¾oz reduced-fat mozzarella cheese, thinly sliced or torn
freshly ground black pepper
45g/1½oz wafer-thin slices lean Parma ham (prosciutto), all visible fat removed
handful of wild rocket (arugula)

Serves 2
Prep: 10 minutes
Cook: 10 minutes

Per serving
300 kcals
Fat: 5.3g
Fibre: 6.5g
Medium GI

Preheat the oven to 230°C/450°F/Gas mark 8. Place a baking sheet in the oven so that it gets really hot.

Spread the passata over the pitta breads right up to the edges, then scatter with pepper strips, onion slices and mushrooms. Arrange the sliced mozzarella over the top.

Place the pittas on the hot baking sheet and cook in the oven for 8–10 minutes until the pitta bases are crisp, the vegetables are softened and the mozzarella has melted.

Remove the pizzas from the oven and grind a little pepper over them. Top with the ham and rocket and serve straight away while they are hot.

OR TRY THIS...
THERE ARE SO MANY TOPPINGS YOU CAN TRY FOR PIZZAS: BE ADVENTUROUS, BUT ALWAYS MAKE SURE YOU USE LOW-CALORIE, LOW-FAT HEALTHY INGREDIENTS. AVOID HOT PEPPERONI SAUSAGE, WHICH HAS 26 CALORIES PER SLICE.

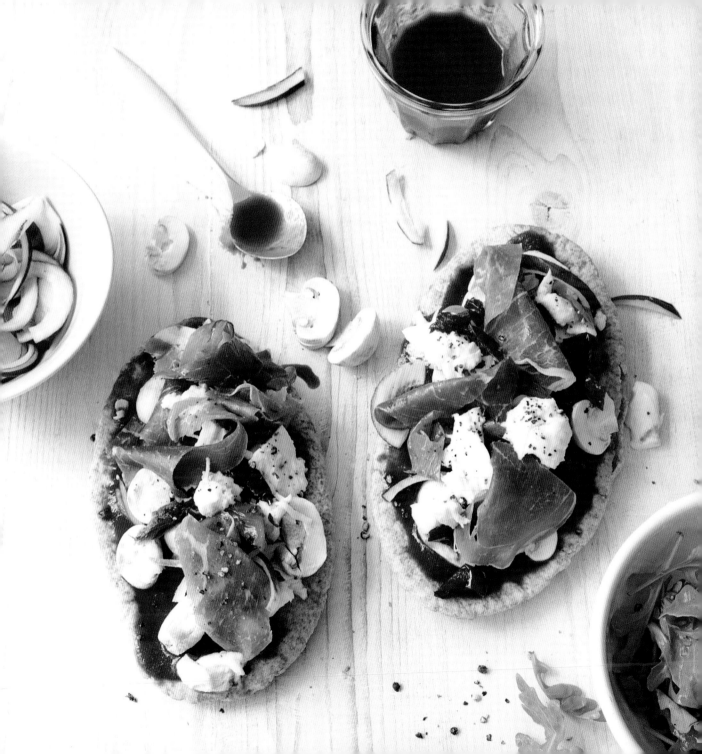

# SIZZLING STEAK FAJITAS

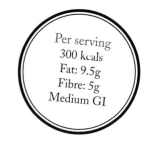

Per serving
300 kcals
Fat: 9.5g
Fibre: 5g
Medium GI

**Fajitas are great finger food and so quick and easy to make. They should be eaten sizzling hot straight from the griddle to be enjoyed at their best. And they are so versatile – you can make them with grilled chicken, large prawns (jumbo shrimp) or as a veggie version with grilled pepper strips and red onions.**

spray oil

1 large red onion, thinly sliced

2 x 100g/3½oz lean, thin-cut sirloin (porterhouse) steaks, all visible fat removed

2 x 35g/1¼oz wholewheat tortillas

few crisp lettuce leaves, sliced

few fresh coriander (cilantro) sprigs, roughly chopped

2 tbsp reduced-fat guacamole

2 tbsp grated reduced-fat Cheddar cheese

**For the hot salsa**

2 large ripe tomatoes, diced

1 hot red chilli, deseeded and diced

¼ red onion, diced

few fresh coriander (cilantro) sprigs, finely chopped

salt and freshly ground black pepper

Serves 2

Prep: 10 minutes

Cook: 10 minutes

Spray a non-stick ridged griddle pan lightly with oil and place over a medium heat. When it's hot, add the onion and cook for 5–10 minutes, turning occasionally, until softened, slightly charred and starting to caramelize.

Push the onion to one side or remove from the pan. Turn up the heat and add the steaks. Cook for 2–4 minutes on each side, depending on how rare or well cooked you like it. Remove from the pan and cut into thin slices.

Put the tortillas in the hot pan – just long enough to warm them through.

Meanwhile, mix all the salsa ingredients together in a bowl.

Arrange the lettuce, coriander, steak and onion on top of the warm tortillas. Add the guacamole and salsa and sprinkle with grated cheese. Roll up and eat immediately.

OR TRY THIS…
INSTEAD OF THE STEAK,. GRILL 250G/9OZ SKINNED CHICKEN BREAST FILLETS, CUT INTO CHUNKS. IT WILL TAKE A LITTLE LONGER TO COOK: KEEP TURNING THE CHICKEN UNTIL IT IS GOLDEN BROWN ALL OVER AND COOKED RIGHT THROUGH AND NO LONGER PINK INSIDE. THE CALORIES WILL STAY THE SAME, BUT THE FAT COUNT WILL BE LOWER: 7G PER SERVING.

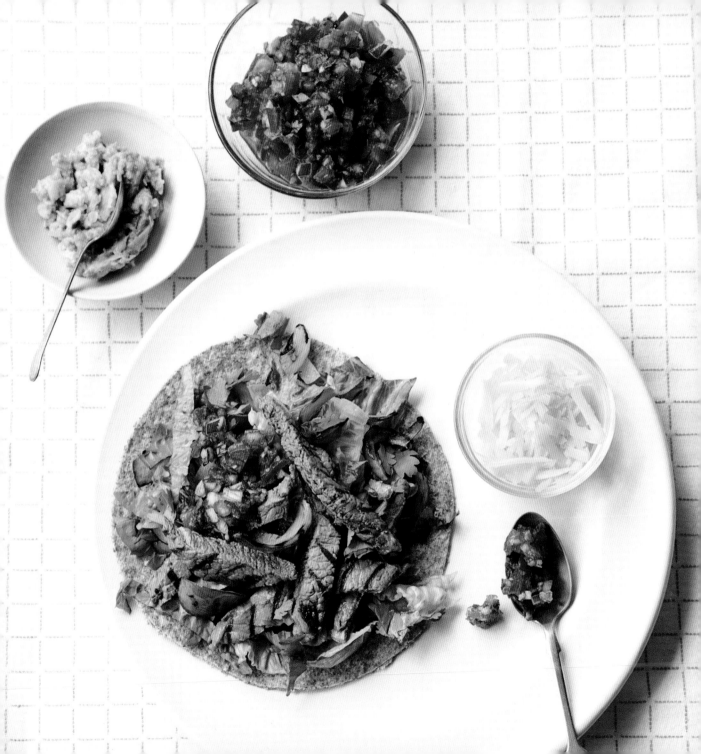

# STEAK GRILL WITH SWEET POTATO 'FRIES'

**Sweet potatoes have more fibre, minerals and less calories than regular potatoes. By cooking sweet potatoes this way, you can continue to enjoy eating 'fries'. These are not only healthier but they also have only a fraction of the calories and fat content of regular French fries! Choose lean steaks and trim off and throw away any visible fat – it can add over 50 calories and 8g fat per steak.**

2 x 125g/4½oz sweet potatoes, peeled and cut lengthways into matchstick 'fries'
spray olive oil
few fresh rosemary sprigs, leaves stripped
few fresh thyme sprigs, leaves picked
freshly ground black pepper
pinch of sea salt crystals
2 x 125g/4½oz lean sirloin (porterhouse) steaks, all visible fat removed
100g/3½oz grilled mushrooms
100g/3½oz grilled cherry tomatoes on the vine

Serves 2
Prep: 10 minutes
Cook: 20–25 minutes

Preheat the oven to 200°C/400°F/Gas mark 6.

Arrange the sweet potatoes 'fries' in a single layer on a non-stick baking tray, spreading them out. Spray lightly with oil and sprinkle with the rosemary and thyme leaves. Grind some pepper over the top and season lightly with sea salt.

Cook in the oven for about 20 minutes, turning the sweet potato occasionally, until it's cooked and tender inside and golden brown and crisp outside.

Meanwhile, lightly spray a non-stick ridged griddle pan with oil and place over a high heat. When the pan is really hot, add the steaks and cook for 2–3 minutes on each side (rare); 4–5 minutes (medium); or 5–6 minutes (well done), depending on how well cooked you like them.

Serve the steaks immediately with the sweet potato 'fries' and some grilled mushrooms and cherry tomatoes.

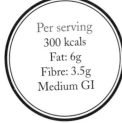

Per serving
300 kcals
Fat: 6g
Fibre: 3.5g
Medium GI

OR TRY THIS...
USE REALLY LEAN RUMP STEAK INSTEAD OF SIRLOIN IF YOU PREFER. THE CALORIES AND FAT GRAMS ARE THE SAME AS LONG AS YOU CAREFULLY REMOVE ALL THE VISIBLE FAT.

# STEAK AND SPINACH TOWERS

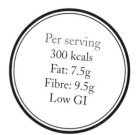

Per serving
300 kcals
Fat: 7.5g
Fibre: 9.5g
Low GI

**The red onion marmalade is delicious and very low in calories (less than 40 calories per serving and only a trace of fat), so you could make double the quantity, set aside to cool and then store in a sealed container in the refrigerator, where it will keep for up to a week. Use it to jazz up grilled chicken or cold meat or as a relish for grilled halloumi cheese.**

350g/12oz baby spinach leaves
1 tablespoon water
good pinch of grated nutmeg
4 tbsp virtually fat-free natural fromage frais
salt and freshly ground black pepper
2 x 100g/3½oz lean beef fillet (tenderloin) steaks, all visible fat removed
spray oil
1 x 150g/5½oz baked jacket potato
snipped fresh chives, to garnish

**For the red onion marmalade**
spray oil
1 red onion, thinly sliced
pinch of brown sugar
1 tsp balsamic vinegar

Serves 2
Prep: 10 minutes
Cook: 25 minutes

Make the red onion marmalade: lightly spray a non-stick frying pan with oil and place over a low heat. Add the sliced onion and cook very gently for about 15 minutes, stirring occasionally, until it's very tender and starting to caramelize. Stir in the sugar and vinegar, season with salt and pepper and cook gently for 10 minutes.

Meanwhile, put the spinach in a large saucepan with the water. Place the pan over a low-medium heat and cover with a lid. Cook for 3–4 minutes, shaking the pan occasionally, until the leaves wilt and turn bright green. Drain well in a colander, pressing down with a saucer to squeeze out any excess moisture. Stir in the grated nutmeg and half the fromage frais. Season to taste and keep warm.

Preheat a ridged griddle pan over a medium-high heat. When it's really hot, season the steaks with pepper, add to the pan and cook for 2–3 minutes on each side (rare); 4–5 minutes (medium); or 5–6 minutes (well done), depending on how well cooked you like them.

Make a neat bed of spinach on each serving plate and place a steak on top. Add a spoonful of warm red onion marmalade on top of each steak. Split the baked potato, top with the remaining fromage frais and the snipped chives and serve immediately.

OR TRY THIS…
OMIT THE BAKED POTATO AND FROMAGE FRAIS AND YOU CAN SERVE THIS AS A 200-CALORIE MEAL.

# QUICK MOUSSAKA

Most moussaka recipes are very rich and are made with a lot of oil as well as a béchamel sauce topping, which add a lot of calories and fat. This speedy version is topped with 0% fat Greek yogurt, which not only reduces the fat and calorie count but also saves time. It's a really healthy dish and tastes just as good as a traditional moussaka.

spray oil
1 large aubergine (eggplant), thinly sliced
1 onion, finely chopped
2 garlic cloves, crushed
125g/4½oz button (white) mushrooms, thinly sliced
225g/8oz extra lean minced (ground) lamb (max 10% fat)
pinch of ground allspice
200g/7oz canned chopped tomatoes
salt and freshly ground black pepper
1 free-range egg
150g/5½oz/⅔ cup 0% fat Greek yogurt
2 tbsp grated reduced-fat Cheddar cheese
100g/3½oz courgettes (zucchini) or baby leeks, pan-grilled, to serve

Serves 2
Prep: 10 minutes
Cook: 35–40 minutes

Preheat the oven to 200°C/400°F/Gas mark 6.

Spray a non-stick frying pan lightly with oil and place over a medium heat. When it's hot, add the aubergine slices and cook until golden brown on both sides. Remove from the pan and set aside on a plate lined with kitchen paper.

Add the onion, garlic and mushrooms to the pan and cook for about 5 minutes until tender and golden.

Add the lamb and spices and cook for 5 minutes, stirring occasionally. Add the canned tomatoes, season to taste, then cook for a further 5 minutes.

Put half the lamb mixture in an ovenproof dish and cover with half the aubergine slices. Add the remaining lamb mixture and then top with the rest of the aubergine.

Whisk the egg and yogurt together in a jug and pour over the aubergine. Season lightly and sprinkle with grated cheese.

Bake in the oven for 15–20 minutes until bubbling and golden brown on top. Serve immediately with pan-grilled courgettes or baby leeks.

OR TRY THIS...
USE 250G/9OZ VERY LEAN MINCED BEEF (LESS THAN 5% FAT) INSTEAD OF LAMB. THE FAT COUNT WILL BE REDUCED TO 9.5G PER SERVING; THE CALORIE COUNT WILL STAY APPROXIMATELY THE SAME.

Per serving
300 kcals
Fat: 10g
Fibre: 5.3g
Medium GI

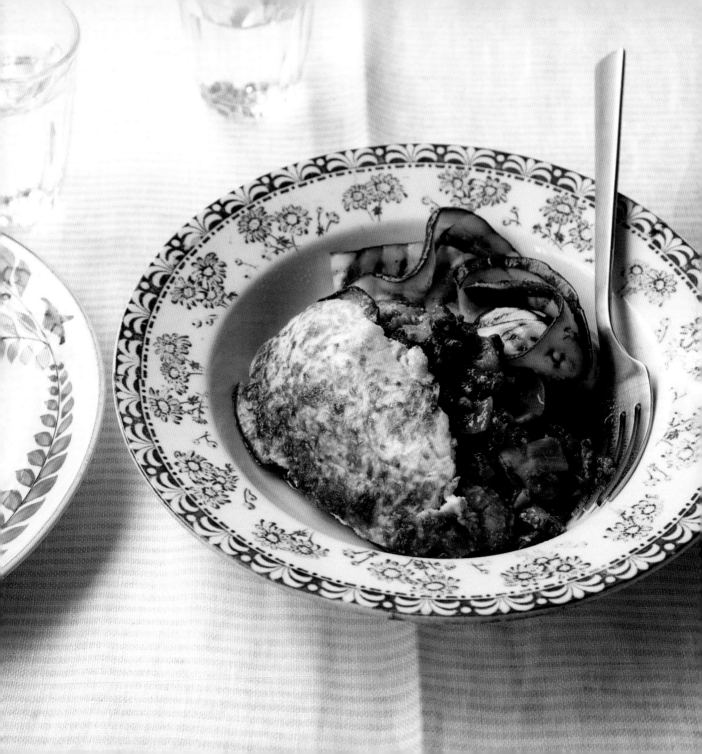

# SPICED LAMB STEAKS WITH QUINOA SALAD

**Quinoa has become a very fashionable grain because it is gluten-free and a complete protein, containing all eight essential amino acids, as well as valuable minerals. The translucent bead-shaped grains have a nutty flavour and firm texture and make a tasty alternative to couscous and bulgur wheat.**

60g/2¼oz/⅓ cup quinoa (dry weight)

grated zest and juice of 1 large lemon

2 spring onions (scallions), finely chopped

1 baby avocado, stoned, peeled and diced

handful of fresh mint, chopped

salt and freshly ground black pepper

1 tsp ground coriander

1 tsp ground cumin

2 x 75g/2¾oz lean lamb steaks, all visible fat removed

spray oil

watercress or wild rocket (arugula), to serve

Serves 2

Prep: 15 minutes

Cook: 10 minutes

Cook the quinoa in a saucepan of boiling water according to the packet instructions. Drain well.

Put the hot quinoa in a bowl with the lemon zest and juice, spring onions, avocado and mint. Add salt to taste and a good grinding of pepper and mix together gently.

Rub the ground spices into both sides of the lamb steaks. Lightly spray a ridged griddle pan with oil and set over a medium-high heat. When it's hot, add the lamb and cook for 3–5 minutes on each side, depending on how pink or well cooked you like your lamb.

Serve the grilled lamb steaks with the quinoa salad and some watercress or rocket.

OR TRY THIS...
GRILLED CHICKEN, STEAKS, PRAWNS (SHRIMP) OR WHITE FISH FILLETS CAN ALL BE SERVED WITH THIS QUINOA SALAD, OR TRY BROCHETTES OF GRILLED VEGETABLES AND HALLOUMI CHEESE.

Per serving
300 kcals
Fat: 13g
Fibre: 3.5g
Low GI

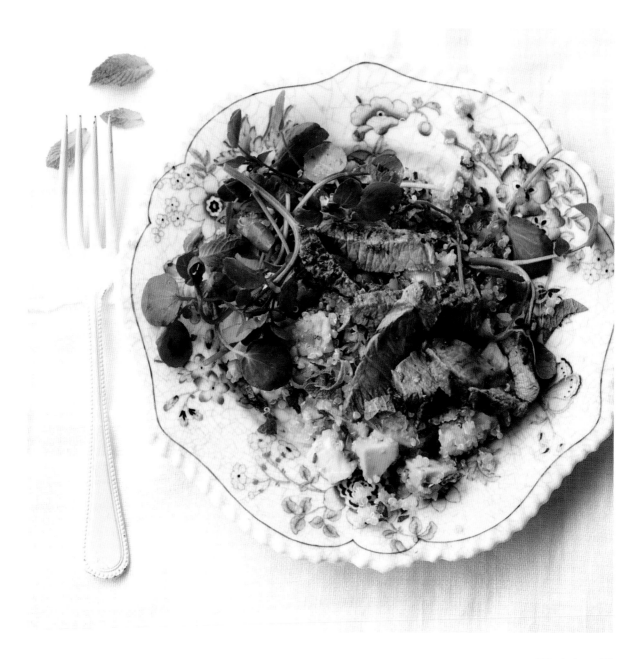

# PORK WITH APRICOT STUFFING

**Pork fillet, also known as tenderloin, is a very lean cut with hardly any fat, making it a great source of protein for slimmers. The sweetness of stone and orchard fruits, especially apricots, plums, apples and pears, complements the flavour perfectly.**

1 x 300g/10½oz lean pork fillet (tenderloin) in one piece, all visible fat removed

2 fresh apricots, halved, stoned and quartered

4 fresh sage leaves

spray olive oil

sea salt flakes and freshly ground black pepper

2 red dessert apples, cored

100ml/3½fl oz/scant ½ cup dry (hard) cider or apple juice

2 tbsp half-fat crème fraîche

Serves 2
Prep: 10 minutes
Cook: 35 minutes

Per serving
300 kcals
Fat: 6g
Fibre: 3g
Medium GI

Preheat the oven to 200°C/400°F/Gas mark 6.

Make a deep slit along one side of the pork with a sharp knife, leaving the ends intact. Push the apricots and sage leaves into the slit. Close the fillet over it and tie with kitchen string to hold the filling securely in place.

Place the pork in a roasting pan, spray lightly with oil and sprinkle some sea salt and pepper over the top. Bake in the oven for 15 minutes.

Score the apples round the middle and put them in the pan with the pork. Pour the cider or apple juice over the top and bake in the oven for a further 15–20 minutes until the pork is thoroughly cooked and the apples are tender.

Remove the pork and apples from the pan and keep warm. Boil the pan juices on top of the stove until they reduce, then stir in the crème fraîche to make a creamy sauce.

Remove the string from the pork and carve into slices. Serve in the creamy sauce with the baked apples.

OR TRY THIS...
IF FRESH APRICOTS ARE UNAVAILABLE OR OUT OF SEASON, USE 20G/¾OZ READY-TO-EAT DRIED APRICOTS INSTEAD. CHOP THEM INTO PIECES AND USE AS A FILLING WITH THE SAGE LEAVES.

# CHICKEN SALTIMBOCCA

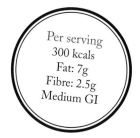

Per serving
300 kcals
Fat: 7g
Fibre: 2.5g
Medium GI

Here's a classic Italian dish, much loved in Rome, where it is traditionally made with veal. Saltimbocca literally means 'jump in the mouth' and this is so succulent that it's almost impossible to resist. You can serve it with boiled or steamed fine green beans – 100g/3½oz will add 12 calories, 0.2g fat and 1.3g fibre per serving.

2 x 100g/3½oz skinless, boneless chicken breasts

4 fresh sage leaves

4 thin slices lean Parma ham (prosciutto), all visible fat removed

spray olive oil

200g/7oz button (white) mushrooms, thinly sliced

200ml/7fl oz/scant 1 cup chicken stock

50ml/2fl oz/scant ¼ cup Marsala

salt and freshly ground black pepper

2 tbsp half-fat crème fraîche

2 tbsp finely chopped fresh parsley

50g/2oz fusilli or fettuccine (dried weight)

Serves 2
Prep: 10 minutes
Cook: 25 minutes

Place each chicken breast between two sheets of greaseproof paper and beat with a rolling pin until it is thin and flat. Place two sage leaves on top of each chicken escalope and then wrap two slices of ham around it.

Lightly spray a frying pan with oil and set over a medium heat. When it's hot, add the chicken and cook for a few minutes until golden brown on both sides.

Add the mushrooms to the pan and cook for 4–5 minutes, stirring occasionally, until lightly browned.

Pour in the chicken stock and Marsala and simmer gently for 10–15 minutes until the chicken is cooked through and the sauce is reduced and syrupy. Season to taste with salt and pepper. Reduce the heat to a bare simmer and stir in the crème fraîche. Heat through very gently without boiling.

While the sauce is cooking, cook the pasta as per the manufacturer's instructions on the packet until *al dente*. Drain well.

Serve the chicken in the sauce, sprinkled with parsley, with the freshly cooked pasta.

OR TRY THIS...
USE TURKEY OR VEAL ESCALOPES INSTEAD OF CHICKEN.
SUBSTITUTE A MEDIUM WHITE WINE FOR THE MARSALA.

# THAI CHICKEN TRAYBAKE

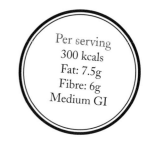

Per serving
300 kcals
Fat: 7.5g
Fibre: 6g
Medium GI

**The great thing about this spicy recipe is that everything is cooked in the same dish, which makes it so easy to prepare and to clean up afterwards. You can buy prepared boned chicken thighs, but you will have to remove the skin and trim away any visible fat. Chicken breasts can be cooked in the same way, but the thigh meat has a more intense flavour.**

4 x 60g/2¼oz skinless, boneless chicken thighs
1 red onion, quartered
1 red (bell) pepper, deseeded and cut into chunks
1 yellow (bell) pepper, deseeded and cut into chunks
150g/5½oz sweet potato, peeled and cut into wedges
spray olive oil
freshly ground black pepper
few fresh coriander sprigs, chopped

**For the Thai paste**
2.5cm/1in piece of fresh root ginger, peeled and chopped
2 garlic cloves, peeled
1 lemongrass stalk, peeled and chopped
1 red chilli, deseeded and diced
grated zest and juice of 1 lime
15g/½oz fresh coriander (cilantro), chopped

Serves 2
Prep: 10 minutes
Cook: 35 minutes

Preheat the oven to 200°C/400°F/Gas mark 6.

Blitz all the Thai paste ingredients together in a blender until you have a smooth paste. Rub this into the chicken thighs.

Arrange the chicken thighs, onion, peppers and sweet potato in an ovenproof dish or roasting pan. Spray lightly with oil and grind some pepper over the top. Bake in the oven for 35 minutes, turning the chicken and vegetables in the pan juices once or twice. Remove from the oven when the chicken is cooked right through and the vegetables are tender.

Divide the chicken and the vegetables between two serving plates and serve immediately with a sprinkling of chopped coriander.

SLIM FACT...
THE THAI PASTE IS SIMPLE TO MAKE AND MUCH LOWER IN FAT AND CALORIES THAN THE READY-MADE GREEN AND RED CURRY PASTES SOLD IN JARS. USE THIS PASTE FOR SMEARING ON CHICKEN BREASTS OR PRAWNS (SHRIMP) BEFORE GRILLING OR BAKING THEM.

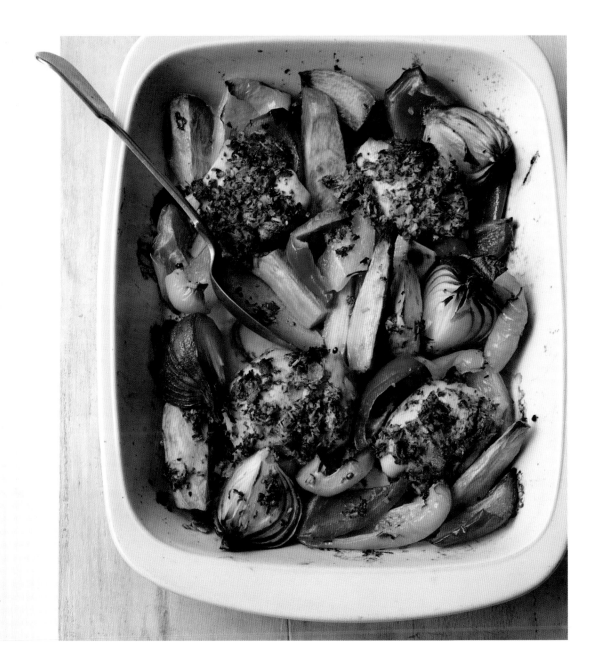

# JAMAICAN JERKED CHICKEN

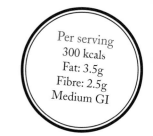

Per serving
300 kcals
Fat: 3.5g
Fibre: 2.5g
Medium GI

You can buy jerk seasoning in small jars in the herbs and spices sections of large supermarkets. If you love hot food, serve the jerked chicken with a dash of West Indian hot pepper sauce – a teaspoon is 3 calories but you won't need that much!

2 x 150g/5½oz skinless, boneless chicken breasts
2 tsp jerk spice seasoning
2 garlic cloves, crushed
grated zest and juice of 1 lime
60g/2¼oz/scant ⅓ cup basmati rice
50g/1¾oz rocket (arugula) or crisp salad leaves
¼ cucumber, diced
few drops of balsamic vinegar

**For the papaya salsa**
100g/3½oz ripe papaya, peeled, deseeded and diced
2 spring onions (scallions), finely chopped
1 red chilli, deseeded and chopped
juice of 1 lime
few fresh coriander (cilantro) sprigs, finely chopped

Serves 2
Prep: 20 minutes
Chill: 1 hour
Cook: 25–30 minutes

Slash each chicken breast two or three times with a sharp knife. Mix the jerk seasoning with the garlic, lime zest and juice in a small bowl. Rub this mixture over the chicken and into the slashes. Cover and leave in the refrigerator or at least 1 hour.

Preheat the oven to 200°C/400°F/Gas mark 6.

Put the chicken in an ovenproof dish and spoon over the jerk mixture. Bake in the oven for 25–30 minutes, or until the chicken is cooked and the juices run clear when it's pierced with a skewer.

While the chicken is cooking, cook the rice according to the packet instructions.

Mix all the papaya salsa ingredients together in a bowl.

Serve the jerked chicken with the cooked rice and salsa, alongside the salad leaves and cucumber drizzled with balsamic vinegar.

OR TRY THIS...
INSTEAD OF BAKING THE CHICKEN IN THE OVEN, COOK IT UNDER A PREHEATED HOT GRILL OR, BETTER STILL, ON A BARBECUE FOR AN AUTHENTIC SMOKY FLAVOUR.

# GREEK-STYLE ROAST CHICKEN

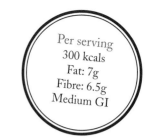

Per serving
300 kcals
Fat: 7g
Fibre: 6.5g
Medium GI

**This is a delicious low-fat way to roast a chicken and it will have a wonderful lemon aroma and flavour. Don't cheat and eat the skin when nobody's looking – it adds a third as much again of the calories in the skinless meat.**

1 x 1.5kg/3lb roasting chicken
salt and freshly ground black pepper
few fresh oregano and thyme sprigs
500g/1lb 2oz Charlotte potatoes, halved or quartered
8 unpeeled garlic cloves (optional)
2 lemons
spray olive oil
4 tbsp water

For the cos lettuce salad
1 cos (romaine) lettuce, separated into leaves
bunch of spring onions (scallions), trimmed and sliced
1 green (bell) pepper, deseeded and thinly sliced
½ cucumber, thinly sliced
3 tbsp oil-free vinaigrette dressing
juice of 1 lemon

Serves 4
Prep: 10 minutes
Cook: 1½ hours

Preheat the oven to 200°C/400°F/Gas mark 6.

Place the chicken in a large roasting pan. Season with salt and pepper and push a few of the herb sprigs inside the cavity. Arrange the potatoes around the chicken and tuck in the unpeeled garlic cloves.

Cut 1 lemon in half and squeeze it over the chicken and potatoes. Place the squeezed halves inside the chicken. Cut the other lemon into wedges and place among the potatoes. Strip the leaves off the remaining herb sprigs and scatter over the top. Lightly spray the chicken and potatoes with oil. Carefully pour the water into a corner of the roasting pan.

Roast in the oven for 1½ hours, basting the chicken occasionally with the pan juices, and turning the potatoes over as they brown. If the potatoes are cooked before the chicken, remove them and keep warm.

Remove the cooked chicken from the oven, cover with foil and set aside to rest for 10 minutes before carving. Meanwhile, mix all the salad ingredients together in a large bowl and season with salt and pepper.

Carve the chicken into slices – allow about 115g/4oz or 3–4 thin slices per person – discarding the skin. Serve with the potatoes, roasted lemon wedges and salad. If wished, you can squeeze the soft garlic out of the skins into the salad.

COOK'S TIP...
TO CHECK IF THE CHICKEN IS COOKED, INSERT A SKEWER OR A THIN-BLADED KNIFE INTO THE MEATY PART OF ONE OF THE THIGHS. IF THE JUICES RUN CLEAR, THE CHICKEN IS READY.

# LEBANESE LEMON AND GARLIC CHICKEN

**In Lebanese households, several lemons would be squeezed over the chicken and potatoes; you can add more lemon juice than the amount suggested below without affecting the overall calorie count.**

1½ large lemons
225g/8oz baby new potatoes, halved
250g/9oz skinless, boneless chicken breasts, cubed
2 garlic cloves, crushed
salt and freshly ground black pepper
2 unpeeled garlic cloves
spray olive oil
good pinch of paprika
a few fresh parsley sprigs, chopped
harissa paste (optional)

*Lebanese salad*
2 ripe juicy tomatoes, chopped
1 yellow (bell) pepper, deseeded and chopped
¼ red onion, chopped
¼ cucumber, cut into chunks
1 small cos (romaine) lettuce, sliced
bunch of mixed fresh herbs, such as mint, parsley, basil, chopped
2 tbsp oil-free vinaigrette dressing
squeeze of lemon juice
few drops of balsamic vinegar

Serves 2
Prep: 10 minutes
Cook: 45 minutes

Preheat the oven to 190°C/375°F/Gas mark 5. Squeeze the juice from 1 lemon and cut the half lemon into slices or wedges.

Put the potatoes and chicken in a shallow ovenproof dish. Sprinkle the crushed garlic, lemon juice and seasoning over the top. Tuck in the garlic cloves and lemon slices. Spray lightly with olive oil and then stir gently until everything is well coated. Dust with paprika and cover the dish with foil.

Bake in the oven for 30 minutes before removing the foil. Return to the oven and cook for a further 15 minutes until the chicken is cooked right through and the potatoes are tender. Sprinkle the parsley over the top.

Meanwhile, make the salad: mix the tomatoes, pepper, onion, cucumber, lettuce and herbs together in a bowl. Shake the vinaigrette, lemon juice and balsamic vinegar together in a screwtop jar until well combined. Toss the salad gently in the dressing.

Divide the chicken and potatoes between two serving plates, squeezing the garlic out of the skins. Serve with the salad and a little harissa, if wished.

Per serving
300 kcals
Fat: 3.8g
Fibre: 6g
Low GI

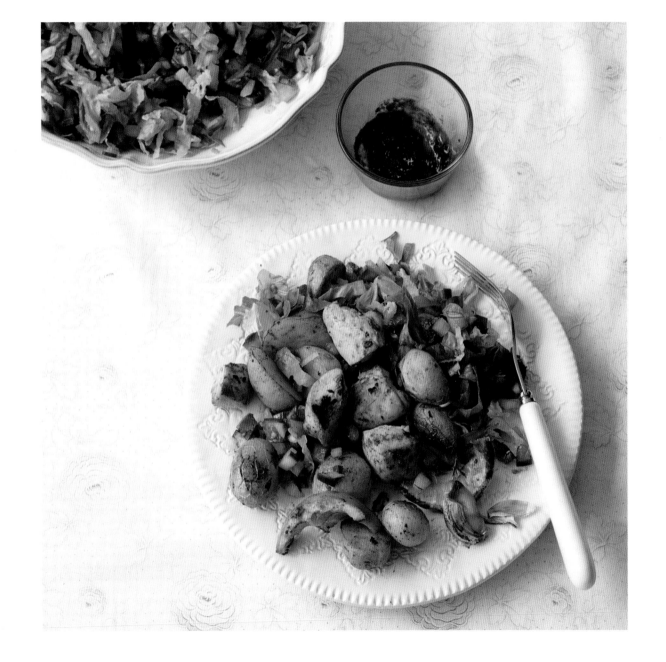

# MALAYSIAN PRAWN LAKSA

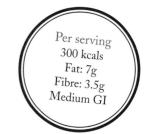

Per serving
300 kcals
Fat: 7g
Fibre: 3.5g
Medium GI

**Laksa is a substantial meal in a bowl. It's quick and easy to make and there's practically no washing-up. Be sure to use reduced-fat coconut milk – it has 70 less calories and 7g fat per 100ml/3½fl oz/scant ½ cup than the whole milk. You can buy it in cans in delis and most supermarkets.**

spray oil
1 onion, chopped
2 garlic cloves, crushed
1 tsp chopped fresh root ginger
1 small red chilli, deseeded and chopped
1 lemongrass stalk, peeled and finely chopped
300ml/½ pint/1¼ cups fish or vegetable stock
juice of 1 lime
100ml/3½fl oz/scant ½ cup reduced-fat coconut milk
100g/3½oz/1 cup bean sprouts
200g/7oz cooked rice noodles
200g/7oz peeled raw tiger prawns (jumbo shrimp)
salt and freshly ground black pepper
2 spring onions (scallions), shredded
few fresh coriander (cilantro) sprigs, roughly chopped

Serves 2
Prep: 15 minutes
Cook: 15 minutes

Lightly spray a large deep frying pan or wok with oil and place over a high heat. When it's hot, add the onion, garlic, ginger, chilli and lemongrass and stir-fry for 2–3 minutes until the onion is golden brown.

Add the stock, lime juice and coconut milk. Reduce the heat and cook gently for 5 minutes, then add the bean sprouts and cooked rice noodles and simmer gently for 5 minutes.

Add the prawns and cook gently for about 3 minutes until they are cooked and pink. Season to taste with salt and pepper.

Ladle the laksa into two deep bowls. Sprinkle with the shredded spring onions and chopped coriander and serve.

OR TRY THIS...
MAKE CHICKEN LAKSA BY ADDING 150G/5½OZ DICED SKINNED CHICKEN BREAST AT THE SAME TIME AS THE STOCK AND COCONUT MILK. COOK AS ABOVE AND OMIT THE PRAWNS. THE CALORIES WILL STAY THE SAME.

# SMOKED FISH AND SPINACH GRATIN

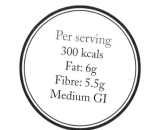

**A perfect supper on a cold evening. It doesn't take long to prepare when you come in from work, and you can relax or get on with your chores while it's cooking. And this is a great low-fat way to make a quick and easy white sauce, which you can also use for macaroni cheese, cauliflower cheese or topping a lasagne.**

450g/1lb baby spinach leaves

175g/6oz tomatoes, peeled and sliced

300g/10½oz leftover cooked smoked haddock or cod fillets, skinned, boned and flaked

3 tbsp chopped fresh parsley

1 tbsp grated Parmesan cheese

15g/½oz/generous ¼ cup fresh white breadcrumbs

**For the white sauce**

1 tbsp cornflour (cornstarch)

150ml/¼ pint/⅔ cup skimmed (lowfat) milk

85g/3oz/generous ⅓ cup virtually fat-free natural fromage frais

pinch of nutmeg

salt and freshly ground black pepper

Serves 2

Prep: 15 minutes

Cook: 30 minutes

Preheat the oven to 200°C/400°C/Gas mark 6.

Put the spinach in a large saucepan set over a very low heat. Cover with a lid and cook, shaking the pan occasionally, for 2–3 minutes until the spinach wilts and turns bright green. Drain thoroughly, pressing down on the spinach with a saucer to squeeze out all the moisture. Chop it finely.

Make the white sauce: blend the cornflour with a little of the cold milk in a bowl. Heat the remaining milk in a small saucepan and bring to the boil. Stir in the cornflour mixture and cook, stirring with a wooden spoon for 1–2 minutes until the sauce is thick and smooth. Remove from the heat and beat in the fromage frais, nutmeg, salt and pepper.

Cover the bottom of a shallow ovenproof dish with overlapping slices of tomato. Spread the spinach over the top and then cover with the flaked smoked haddock.

Stir the parsley into the white sauce and pour over the haddock. Sprinkle the grated Parmesan and breadcrumbs over the top. Cook in the oven for 20 minutes until bubbling, crisp and golden brown. Serve hot.

OR TRY THIS…
IF YOU DON'T HAVE ANY LEFTOVER SMOKED FISH, COOK RAW FILLETS BY SIMMERING THEM GENTLY IN A FRYING PAN OR WIDE SAUCEPAN OF WATER OVER A LOW HEAT FOR ABOUT 10 MINUTES. DRAIN AND PICK THEM OVER FOR ANY BONES, THEN BREAK INTO LARGE FLAKES.

# RED MULLET
# WITH PESTO SAUCE

**Red mullet are delicious, especially on a warm summer's evening. You can use 2 x 150g/5oz sea bass fillets instead and cook them in the same way. The calories will stay the same, but the fat grams per serving will be 0.5g less. If you can buy only whole red mullet, ask the fishmonger to fillet them for you.**

4 x 75g/2¾oz red mullet fillets
(with skin)
salt and freshly ground black pepper
spray oil
2 x 80g/2¾oz cherry tomatoes on the
vine
few fresh chives, to garnish
lemon wedges, to serve

**For the lemony pesto sauce**
1 tbsp pine nuts
15g/½oz fresh basil leaves
60ml/2fl oz/¼ cup vegetable stock
2 tbsp grated Parmesan cheese
1 tsp olive oil
1 garlic clove, crushed
good squeeze of lemon juice

Serves 2
Prep: 15 minutes
Cook: 10 minutes

Make the pesto: put the pine nuts in a small saucepan and place over a medium heat. Cook, shaking the pan often, for 2–3 minutes until they are toasted and golden. Remove from the pan and leave to cool.

Put the pine nuts, basil, stock, grated Parmesan cheese, olive oil, garlic and lemon juice in a blender and blitz until smooth. The sauce should be quite thick. Cover and chill until ready to eat.

Season the red mullet with salt and pepper. Spray a non-stick frying pan lightly with oil and place over a high heat. Place the mullet, skin-side down, in the hot pan and cook for 2–3 minutes until the skin is crisp and golden. Turn the fillets over and cook for 2–3 minutes on the other side.

While the fish are cooking, cook the tomatoes on the vine in a ridged griddle pan or under a preheated hot grill, until the skins are a little blackened.

Serve the red mullet with the lemony pesto sauce, grilled tomatoes and lemon wedges, and garnish with chives.

Per serving
300 kcals
Fat: 12.5g
Fibre: 1g
Low GI

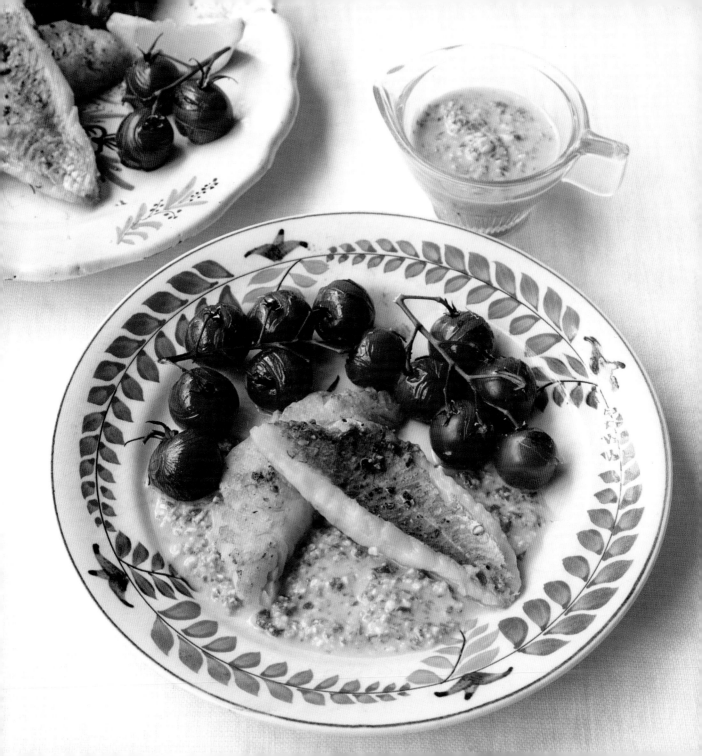

# FISH FILLETS WITH CRISP PARMESAN CRUST

**White fish fillets are low in calories and fat, and can be simply grilled and served with a squeeze of lemon juice and a grinding of black pepper. Adding a crisp cheesy crust makes them more appetizing and takes very little time when you're creating a meal in a hurry.**

30g/1oz/½ cup fresh white breadcrumbs

30g/1oz/generous ¼ cup grated Parmesan cheese

3 tbsp chopped fresh parsley

freshly ground black pepper

pinch of paprika

2 x 150g/5½oz white fish fillets, such as cod or haddock, skinned

spray oil

100g/3½oz baby leaf salad

150g/5½oz tomatoes, diced

1 tbsp capers

2 tbsp oil-free vinaigrette dressing

few fresh basil leaves, torn

Serves 2
Prep: 10 minutes
Cook: 15 minutes

Per serving
300 kcals
Fat: 7g
Fibre: 2g
Low GI

Preheat the oven to 190°C/375°F/Gas mark 5.

In a shallow dish, mix together the breadcrumbs, grated Parmesan, parsley, black pepper and paprika.

Lightly spray the fish fillets with oil and dip them into the seasoned breadcrumbs until they are evenly coated all over. Place them in an ovenproof dish.

Cook in the oven for 15 minutes until the coating is crisp and golden and the fish is cooked through.

Toss the baby salad leaves with the tomatoes, capers, vinaigrette dressing and basil. Serve the piping hot fish fillets immediately with the salad.

OR TRY THIS...
INSTEAD OF USING OIL-FREE VINAIGRETTE FOR DRESSING SALADS, YOU CAN DRIZZLE SOME GOOD-QUALITY BALSAMIC VINEGAR OVER THE TOP. ITS NATURAL SWEETNESS ENHANCES MOST SALAD LEAVES AND VEGETABLES.

# SOY SALMON AND VEGETABLE PARCELS

**Nothing could be simpler than this refreshing, healthy dish – everything is cooked en papillote (in a paper parcel) in the oven, so the fish stays moist and succulent. Salmon is an oily fish and higher in calories and fat than white fish, but because it's so filling you don't need so much. It's also a great source of omega-3 fatty acids, which are good for your heart. Other good sources are mackerel, herring, tuna and sardines.**

2 carrots
2 celery sticks, chopped
4 spring onions (scallions), chopped
1 tsp finely chopped fresh root ginger
grated zest of 1 small lemon
4 star anise
2 x 100g/3½oz salmon fillets, skinned
few fresh coriander (cilantro) sprigs, chopped
salt and freshly ground black pepper
2 tbsp vegetable or fish stock
1 tbsp light soy sauce
50g/1¾oz/¼ cup basmati rice

Serves 2
Prep: 15 minutes
Cook: 15 minutes

Preheat the open to 190°C/375°F/Gas mark 5.

Using a potato peeler, cut the carrots into very thin strips. Divide them between two large squares of greaseproof paper or baking parchment, then add the celery, spring onions, ginger, lemon zest and star anise.

Place the salmon fillets on top and sprinkle with the coriander. Season lightly with salt and pepper and drizzle over the stock and soy sauce.

Fold the paper over the salmon and vegetables, twisting the ends securely together to make two sealed parcels. Place them on a baking sheet and cook in the oven for 15 minutes until the vegetables are tender and the salmon is cooked right through.

Meanwhile, cook the rice according to the packet instructions.

Transfer the salmon and vegetables to two serving plates and serve immediately with the hot rice.

Per serving
300 kcals
Fat: 11.5g
Fibre: 2.5g
Medium GI

# TEX-MEX VEGGIE BURGERS

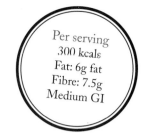

Per serving
300 kcals
Fat: 6g fat
Fibre: 7.5g
Medium GI

**These burgers are a great way of using up leftover cooked rice, whether it's white or brown. They taste great served with low-fat guacamole, but remember that a tablespoon will add 22 calories and 2g fat.**

1 x 200g/7oz can sweetcorn kernels
½ red onion, finely chopped
1 small red (bell) pepper, deseeded and finely diced
115g/4oz leftover boiled rice
grated zest of 1 lime
1 fresh red chilli, deseeded and finely chopped
2 tbsp chopped fresh coriander (cilantro)
salt and freshly ground black pepper
1 small egg, beaten (optional)
spray oil

For the salad
1 small packet of baby salad leaves
few fresh coriander (cilantro) sprigs, chopped
2 ripe tomatoes, chopped
1 tbsp oil-free vinaigrette dressing

To serve
60g/2¼oz reduced-fat tomato salsa
60g/2¼oz/¼ cup virtually fat-free natural fromage frais

Serves 4
Prep: 15 minutes
Chill: 20 minutes
Cook: 20–25 minutes

Drain the sweetcorn kernels and reserve the liquid. Blitz the sweetcorn to a purée in a blender or food processor for a few seconds.

Put the puréed sweetcorn in a saucepan with the onion, red pepper and reserved liquid. Cover the pan and simmer over a low heat, stirring occasionally, for 10–15 minutes until the mixture has reduced and thickened and the onion and pepper have softened.

Stir in the rice, lime zest, half of the chilli (reserve the rest for the salad dressing) and the coriander. Season to taste with salt and pepper and transfer to a bowl. Cover and chill in the refrigerator for 20 minutes.

Preheat the grill (broiler). Divide the mixture into four portions. Using your hands, shape each one into a round patty. If the mixture is too crumbly, stir in some beaten egg to bind everything together.

Lightly spray the burgers on both sides with oil and cook under the hot grill for 4–5 minutes on each side until crisp and golden brown.

Mix the salad leaves, coriander and tomatoes in a bowl. Combine the vinaigrette dressing with the reserved chopped chilli in a small bowl and then pour over the salad and toss gently. Serve the burgers hot with the salad and a portion of tomato salsa and fromage frais.

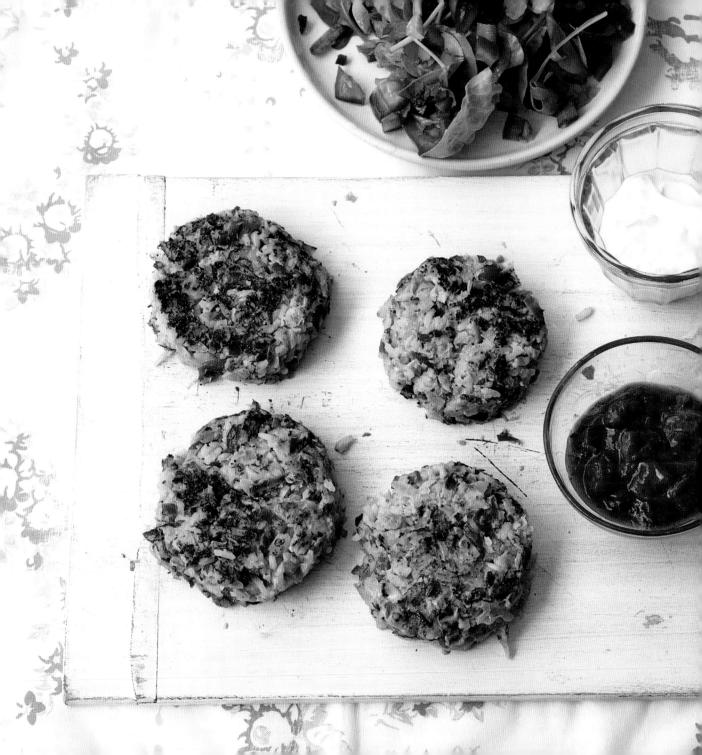

# ROASTED VEGETABLE AND MOZZARELLA BAKE

**This simple supper is wholesome and surprisingly filling. You can make it more substantial if you serve it with cooked pasta, such as fusilli or shells, but this will add 100 calories and 0.5g fat per 85g/3oz (cooked weight) portion, making it a 400-calorie meal.**

1 yellow (bell) pepper, deseeded and cut into chunks

1 red onion, cut into 8 wedges

200g/7oz sweet potato, peeled and cut into chunks

1 small aubergine (eggplant), cut into chunks

few fresh thyme sprigs, leaves picked

spray olive oil

sea salt and freshly ground black pepper

1 x 200g/7oz can chopped tomatoes

150g/5½oz spinach, roughly shredded

100g/3½oz reduced-fat mozzarella cheese, cubed

Serves 2
Prep: 10 minutes
Cook: 50 minutes

Preheat the oven to 200°C/400°F/Gas mark 6.

Put the yellow pepper, onion, sweet potato and aubergine in a large roasting pan. Sprinkle with the thyme leaves, spray lightly with oil and grind some sea salt and black pepper over the top.

Roast in the oven for about 25 minutes, turning the vegetables occasionally, until they are tender and just starting to char.

Put the chopped tomatoes and spinach in a saucepan and heat through gently over a low heat for about 2–3 minutes until the spinach starts to wilt.

Spoon a layer of roasted vegetables into an ovenproof dish, approximately 23 x 13cm/ 9 x 5in. Cover with some of the tomato and spinach mixture and continue layering in this way. Scatter the mozzarella over the top.

Cook in the oven for 15 minutes until the mozzarella has melted. Serve immediately.

Per serving
300 kcals
Fat: 6g
Fibre: 9.5g
Medium GI

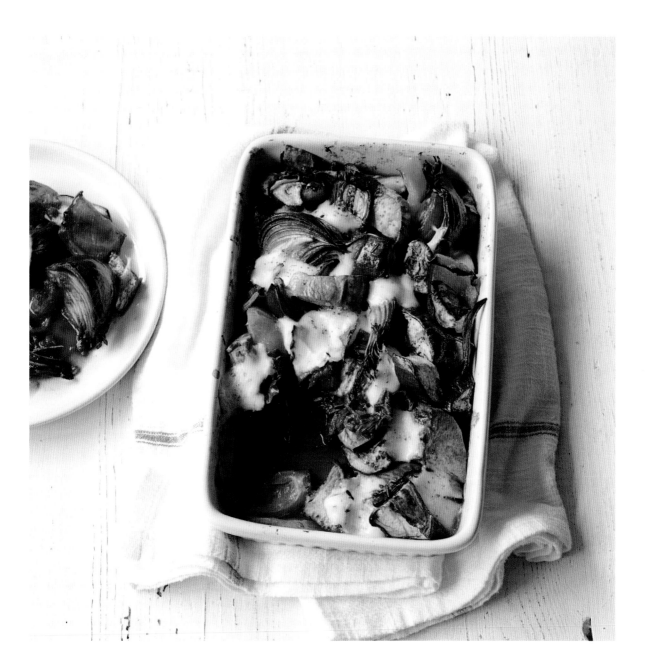

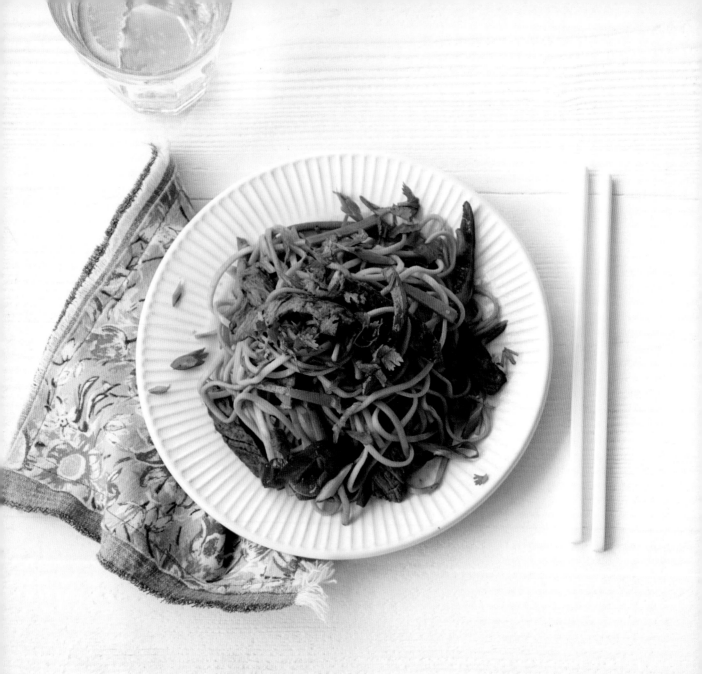

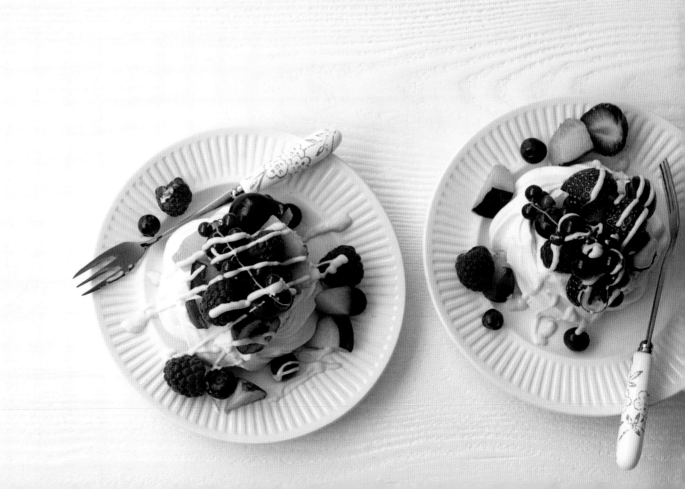

# Index

**apricots**
fruity filo stacks 56
pork with apricot stuffing 154
Asian salad dressing 22
**asparagus**
barbecued Quorn and asparagus salad 86
grilled Californian shrimp salad 42
spring green prawn parcels 52
warm crunchy salad with prawns 77
**aubergines**
quick moussaka 150
Spanish summer bake 94
Thai prawn and aubergine curry 102

**bacon**
all-day breakfast omelette 69
breakfast BLT toastie 66
warm salad with scallop and rocket 80
**bananas**
Baileys banoffee custard 112
kickstart banana berry smoothie 29
**beans**
chunky minestrone 53
Mexican beef salsa pot 92
pan-seared cod with butter beans 100
refried bean tortilla wraps 88
spiced squash and butter bean soup 50
spicy black bean soup 120
**beef**
grilled spiced beef with tabbouleh 129
hot and sour beef salad 83
Mexican beef salsa pot 92
sizzling steak fajitas 146
steak and spinach towers 149
steak grill with sweet potato 'fries' 148
stir-fried chilli beef 125

**bread**
breakfast BLT toastie 66
chicken, mozzarella and pepper quesadillas 140
cinnamon French toast with berries 64
Mexican chicken tortilla baskets 78
quick Parma ham and rocket pizzas 144
refried bean tortilla wraps 88
scrambled egg and pesto tortilla wraps 143
sizzling steak fajitas 146
souvlaki pittas 142
tandoori chicken wraps 87
**bulgur wheat**
grilled spiced beef with tabbouleh 129
Lebanese stuffed pepper rolls 36
salad with roasted vegetables 138
**butternut squash**
baked cheesy stuffed squash 44
spiced squash and butter bean soup 50
spiced tofu and veggie skewers 45
warm roasted squash and lentil salad 130

cabbage, spicy winter coleslaw 48
**cheese**
baked cheesy stuffed squash 44
chicken, mozzarella and pepper quesadillas 140
chicory, pear and Roquefort salad 84
Greek grilled halloumi and vegetables 135
grilled vegetable and halloumi stacks 96
Italian lentil and mozzarella salad 136
Italian portobello mushroom melts 35
mozzarella chicken parcels 90
Mykonos horiatiki salad 49
quick Parma ham and rocket pizzas 144
roasted squash and lentil salad 130

roasted vegetable and mozzarella bake 170
scrambled egg and pesto tortilla wraps 143
**chicken**
Baja griddled chicken salad 139
chicken, mozzarella and pepper quesadillas 140
chicken saltimbocca 155
Greek-style roast 159
hot and sour chicken soup 54
Indonesian chicken satay 40
Jamaican jerked 158
Lebanese lemon and garlic 160
lemon chicken kebabs 91
Mexican chicken tortilla baskets 78
mozzarella chicken parcels 90
spiced buffalo wings 41
tandoori chicken wraps 87
Thai chicken traybake 156
**chickpeas**
chickpea mash and veggie dippers 37
Greek grilled halloumi and vegetables 135
**chicory**
grilled Californian shrimp salad 42
pear and Roquefort salad 84
**chocolate**
frozen berries with white chocolate 60
fruity filo parcels 107
no-cook cake 113
**cod**
grilled with lentils 99
pan-seared with butter beans 100
coleslaw, spicy winter 48
**courgettes**
lemony primavera risotto 128
spring green prawn parcels 52
tomato and rocket frittata 76
**crab**
Maryland crabcakes 103
noodles with spiced crab and lemon 124
**cucumber**
Mykonos horiatiki salad 49
tzatziki 23

**curry**
Malaysian prawn laksa 162
Thai prawn and aubergine curry 102

**desserts**
affogato al caffe 59
amaretti summer fruit meringue 58
apple and blackberry strudel 110
Baileys banoffee custard 112
chocolate fruity filo parcels 107
frozen berries with white chocolate 60
fruity filo stacks 56
no-cook cake 113
summer fruit mini pavlovas 108
tiramisu 109

**eggs**
all-day breakfast omelette 69
cinnamon French toast 64
Mediterranean no-pastry quiches 38
scrambled egg and pesto tortilla wraps 143
scrambled egg and smoked salmon mini blinis 28
Spanish baked eggs with chorizo 118
Spanish roasted pepper and spinach tortilla 132
tomato and rocket frittata 76
tuna eggs Benedict 117

**fish**
fillets with crisp Parmesan crust 166
grilled cod and lentils 99
pan-seared cod with butter beans 100
red mullet with pesto sauce 164
scrambled egg and smoked salmon mini blinis 28
smoked fish and spinach gratin 163
smoked salmon fishcakes 104
soy salmon and vegetable parcels 167
tuna eggs Benedict 117
fruit *see also* specific fruit
amaretti summer fruit meringue 58

174

chocolate fruity filo parcels 107
cinnamon French toast with
    berries 64
exotic fruit salsa 23
filo stacks 56
frozen berries with white
    chocolate 60
granola berry breakfast bowl 67
hi-fibre breakfast muffins 26
porridge with fruit compôte
    116
summer fruit mini pavlovas 108

ham, quick Parma ham and rocket
    pizzas 144
honey mustard dip 41

lamb
    quick moussaka 150
    souvlaki pittas 142
    spiced lamb steaks with quinoa
        salad 152
lentils
    grilled cod and lentils 99
    Indian spiced dhal soup 70
    Italian lentil and mozzarella
        salad 136
    salad with roasted squash 130

muffins
    hi-fibre breakfast muffins 26
    tuna eggs Benedict 117
mushrooms
    all-day breakfast omelette 69
    chicken saltimbocca 155
    hot and sour chicken soup 54
    Italian portobello mushroom
        melts 35
    warm salad with rocket 91

noodles
    Malaysian prawn laksa 162
    stir-fried chilli beef 125
    Thai prawn and vegetable soup
        122

onions
    French onion soup 121
    Mediterranean no-pastry
        quiches 38
    red onion marmalade 149

Parma ham and rocket pizzas 144

pasta
    noodles with spiced crab and
        lemon 124
    prawn and rocket linguine 74
    spring vegetable lasagne stacks
        126
peppers (bell)
    chicken, mozzarella and pepper
        quesadillas 140
    grilled Californian shrimp salad
        42
    Lebanese stuffed pepper rolls
        36
    Mediterranean no-pastry
        quiches 38
    Mykonos horiatiki salad 49
    Spanish baked eggs with chorizo
        118
    Spanish roasted pepper and
        spinach tortilla 132
    Spanish summer bake 94
pesto dip 32
pesto fromage frais 22
pesto veggie mini tartlets 33
pizza, quick Parma ham and
    rocket 144
pork, with apricot stuffing 154
porridge with fruit compôte 116
potatoes
    all-day breakfast omelette 69
    Greek-style roast chicken 159
    Lebanese lemon and garlic
        chicken 160
    smoked salmon fishcakes 104
    Spanish roasted pepper and
        spinach tortilla 132
    Spanish summer bake 94
prawns
    Caesar salad 134
    grilled Californian shrimp salad
        42
    Malaysian laksa 162
    prawn and rocket linguine 74
    spring green prawn parcels 52
    Thai curry with aubergine 102
    Thai skewers 98
    Thai soup with vegetables 122
    warm crunchy asparagus and
        prawn salad 77

quiche, no-pastry 38
quinoa, spiced lamb steaks with
    quinoa salad 152

Quorn, barbecued, with asparagus
    salad 86
refried bean tortilla wraps 88
rice
    Jamaican jerked chicken 158
    lemony primavera risotto 128
    Tex-Mex veggie burgers 168

salad dressings 21, 22, 134
salads
    Baja griddled chicken 139
    barbecued Quorn and asparagus
        86
    bulgur wheat with roasted
        vegetables 138
    chicory, pear and Roquefort 84
    crunchy asparagus and prawn
        77
    griddled hot squid 82
    hot and sour beef 83
    Italian lentil and mozzarella
        136
    Lebanese 160
    Mykonos horiatiki 49
    prawn Caesar 134
    roasted squash and lentil 130
    rocket and mushroom 91
    scallop, bacon and rocket 80
    Spanish roasted vegetable 46
    spiced lamb steaks with quinoa
        152
    spicy winter coleslaw 48
    tomato and basil 103
salmon
    scrambled egg and smoked
        salmon mini blinis 28
    smoked salmon fishcakes 104
    soy salmon and vegetable parcels
        167
sauces
    exotic fruit salsa 23
    low-fat tomato salsa 22
    low-fat white sauce 21
    mint raita 87
    tomato 94
scallops, warm salad with bacon
    and rocket 80
smoothie, kickstart banana berry
    29
soup
    chunky minestrone 53
    French onion 121

hot and sour chicken 54
Indian spiced dhal 70
pumpkin with tortilla chips 72
spiced winter roots 71
spicy black bean 120
Thai prawn and vegetable 122
spinach
    smoked fish and spinach gratin
        163
    Spanish roasted pepper and
        spinach tortilla 132
    steak and spinach towers 149
squid, griddled hot squid salad 82
sweet potato
    spiced wedges 30
    steak grill with sweet potato
        'fries' 148

tabbouleh, with grilled spiced
    beef 129
tartlets, pesto veggie 33
Tex-Mex veggie burgers 168
tofu, spiced tofu and veggie
    skewers 45
tomatoes
    all-day breakfast omelette 69
    frittata with rocket 76
    Mediterranean no-pastry
        quiches 38
    Mykonos horiatiki salad 49
    salad with basil 103
    sauce 94
    Spanish baked eggs with chorizo
        118

vegetables see also salads; specific
    vegetables
    crunchy croquettes 95
    roasted vegetable and mozzarella
        bake 170
    rosemary-skewered vegetables
        32

white sauce, low-fat 21

yogurt
    fruity filo stacks 56
    granola berry breakfast bowl 67
    kickstart banana berry smoothie
        29
    mint raita 87
    salad dressing 21
    spicy winter coleslaw 48
    tzatziki 23

First published in the United Kingdom in 2015
by Pavilion
1 Gower Street, London WC1E 6HD

Copyright © Pavilion Books Company Ltd 2015
Text copyright © Heather Thomas 2015
Photography copyright © Pavilion Books Company Ltd 2015

ISBN: 9781909815902

A CIP catalogue record for this book is available from
the British Library.

10 9 8 7 6 5 4 3 2 1

Reproduction by Rival Colour Ltd, UK
Printed and bound by 1010 Printing International Ltd, China

This book can be ordered direct from the publisher at
www.pavilionbooks.com

Commissioning editor: Fiona Holman
Designer: Laura Russell
Photographer: Clare Winfield
Home economists: Sara Lewis and Valerie Berry
Stylist: Jo Harris

**Heather Thomas** is a cookery writer, editor and the author
of several best-selling cookery, healthy eating, slimming,
and fitness books.

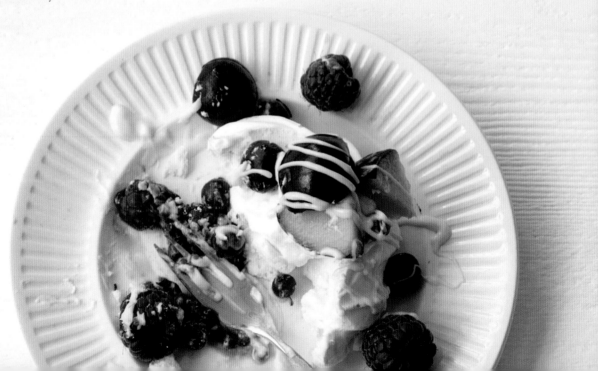